Adrenal cancer

ISBN 2-7420-0593-5

Éditions John Libbey Eurotext
127, avenue de la République
92120 Montrouge, France
Tel: (+33) 01 46 73 06 60
e-mail: contact@jle.com
http://www.jle.com

Editor: Maud Thévenin

© Éditions John Libbey Eurotext, 2006

It is prohibited to reproduce this work or any part of it without authorisation of the publisher or of the Centre Français d'Exploitation du Droit de Copie (CFC), 20, rue des Grands-Augustins, 75006 Paris.

Adrenal cancer

Xavier Bertagna
Endocrine and Metabolic Diseases, Cochin Hospital, APHP, Faculty of Medicine René Descartes, Univ. Paris 5
INSERM U567 and CNRS UMR 8104, Cochin Institute, Paris
Reference Center for Rare Adrenal Gland Diseases
COMETE and ENS@T Clinical Research Networks

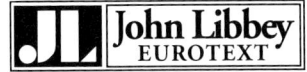

List of contributors

Gwenaelle Abiven, Endocrine and Metabolic Diseases, Cochin Hospital, Paris.

Jérôme Bertherat, INSERM U567 and CNRS UMR 8104, Cochin Institute, Paris; Endocrine and Metabolic Diseases, Cochin Hospital, APHP, Univ. Paris 5, Reference Center for Rare Adrenal Gland Diseases.

Pierre-François Bougnères, Pediatric Endocrinology, Saint Vincent de Paul Hospital, Faculty of Medicine René Descartes, Univ. Paris 5.

Thiery de Baere, Radiology Department, Gustave Roussy Institute, Villejuif.

Bertrand Dousset, Department of Digestive and Endocrine Surgery, Cochin Hospital, Paris, Univ. Paris 5, APHP.

Christine Gicquel, Functional Investigation Department, A. Trousseau Hospital, Paris.

François Goldwasser, Medical Oncology and Internal Medicine Department, Cochin Hospital, Paris.

Lionel Groussin, INSERM U567 and CNRS UMR 8104, Cochin Institute, Paris; Endocrine and Metabolic Diseases, Cochin Hospital, APHP, Univ. Paris 5, Reference Center for Rare Adrenal Gland Diseases.

Paul Legmann, Radiology Department, Cochin Hospital, Faculty of Medicine René Descartes, Univ. Paris 5.

Rossella Libé, INSERM U567 and CNRS UMR 8104, Cochin Institute, Paris; Endocrine and Metabolic Diseases, Cochin Hospital, APHP, Univ. Paris 5, Reference Center for Rare Adrenal Gland Diseases.

Stéphane Silvera, Radiology Department, Cochin Hospital, Faculty of Medicine René Descartes, Univ. Paris 5.

Florence Tenenbaum, Nuclear Medicine, Cochin Hospital, Paris.

Cécile Thomas-Teinturier, Pediatric Endocrinology, Saint Vincent de Paul Hospital, Faculty of Medicine René Descartes, Univ. Paris 5.

Frédérique Tissier, Pathological Anatomy, Cochin Hospital, APHP, Paris; Faculty of Medicine René Descartes, Univ. Paris 5, Paris; Endocrinology Department, INSERM U567, Cochin Institute, Paris.

Contents

Foreword VII

Adrenal cortical carcinoma: clinical management 1
  Xavier Bertagna, Lionel Groussin, Gwenaelle Abiven, Jérôme Bertherat

Molecular genetics of adrenal cortical carcinoma 13
  Rossella Libé, Christine Gicquel, Xavier Bertagna, Jérôme Bertherat

Pathological pattern of adrenal cortical carcinoma 25
  Frédérique Tissier

Imaging in adrenal cortical carcinoma 45
  Paul Legmann, Stéphane Silvera

Chemotherapy of adrenal cortical carcinoma 59
  François Goldwasser, Xavier Bertagna

Surgical treatment of adrenal cortical carcinoma 71
  Bertrand Dousset, Sébastien Gaujoux, Jean-Marc Thillois

Local treatment of adrenal cortical carcinoma metastases with interventional radiology techniques 97
  Thiery de Baere

Scintigraphic explorations in adrenal cortical carcinomas 107
  Florence Tenenbaum

Adrenal cortical tumors in childhood 119
  Cécile Thomas-Teinturier, Pierre-François Bougnères

Foreword

This book on **"Adrenal Cancer"** actually deals with adrenal cortical cancer (it does not address malignant pheochromocytomas).

This is a rare disease, which is often diagnosed at a late stage, and for which there is no totally efficacious medical treatment. Hence, its dismal prognosis.

There are three important messages that the reader should keep in mind after careful reading of all nine chapters:

– **The single best likelihood of "cure"** is when a localized tumor can be subjected to "complete" surgical removal. An early diagnosis is crucial. When faced with an adrenal tumor, an endocrinologist must always ask two questions: could it be a pheochromocytoma? Could it be an adrenal cortical carcinoma? In both cases, it can be a vital question which can make the difference between a fatal issue or cure!

– **Research**, both basic and clinical, is key to further progress: a better understanding of the biology of these tumors has already shed some light on the role of signalling pathways, on some familial syndromes, on new prognostic markers. There is some hope that these approaches will provide us with targeted therapies. Alternatively, progress in our understanding on the general mechanisms of tumor growth might help us design new therapeutic tools using antiangiogenic agents and/or immunotherapy.

– **Reference Centers and National (and European) Networks** are essential to optimize individual patient management, as well as to organize basic research and multicenter clinical trials on this rare disease. For an individual patient, difficult therapeutical options are best offered by a multidisciplinary team (endocrinologist, oncologist, surgeon, radiologist, pathologist, radiotherapist...). In order to boost scientific exchange, to facilitate and harmonize analyses of biological samples, to allow the design of epidemiologic studies or prospective therapeutic trials, several European countries have developed National Networks dedicated to the study of adrenal tumors: COMETE in France, NISGAT in Italy, GANIMED in Germany. In a recent initiative, supported by the Appel d'Offres GIS-Maladies Rares, these national networks have merged into the European network **ENS@T** (**E**uropean **N**etwork for the **S**tudy of **@**drenal **T**umors): its goal is to create a Network wide enough to allow the recruitment of a greater number of patients with rare diseases, and to harmonize diagnostic and therapeutic procedures at the European level. There is strong hope that ENS@T, particularly through its Working Group on Adrenal Cortical Cancer, will sucessfully contribute to the fight against this killer disease.

Adrenal cortical carcinoma: clinical management

Xavier Bertagna, Lionel Groussin, Gwenaelle Abiven, Jérôme Bertherat

APHP, Cochin Hospital, Endocrine and Metabolic Diseases;
Reference Center for Rare Adrenal Gland Diseases;
Endocrinology Department, Institut Cochin; INSERM U567, Faculty of Medicine René Descartes, Univ. Paris 5

Adrenal cortical carcinoma (ACC) is a rare disease with dismal prognosis (Luton, 1990; Wajchenberg, 2000; Allolio, 2004). The single best prognostic factor is when a "localized" (stage 1,2) tumor can be subjected to "complete" removal ("curative" surgery), hence the critical importance of early diagnosis.

There is no medical treatment that has convincingly been shown to provide a definitive solution in advanced (locally invasive and/or metastatic, stage 3,4) ACCs (Schteingart, 2005). O,p'DDD (Mitotane or Lysodren®) has shown some benefit in a minority of patients, and only for brief periods. In this situation a multidisciplinary approach with endocrinologists, surgeons, radiologists, radiotherapists and oncologists is necessary to control hypersecretion, precisely assess tumor extent, and propose possible local actions and/or new chemotherapeutic regimens.

Epidemiology

A rare disease, the estimated incidence of ACC is about 1-2 per million and per year (Wajchenberg, 2000). Age distribution shows two peaks, the first occurring in early childhood (see chapter 9 by Teinturier), and the second between 40 and 50 years. There is a slightly higher female ratio.

Although most ACCs are of sporadic origin, they may also be part of congenital and/or familial diseases (see chapter 2 by Bertherat).

The Wiedeman-Beckwith syndrome (11p15 locus) and the Li-Fraumeni syndrome (p53 at 17p13 locus) are both associated with the development of hereditary tumors, including ACCs. The Multiple Endocrine Neoplasia type 1 (MEN 1) typically associates tumors of the parathyroid glands, the pancreas and the pituitary; in about 30% of patients, adrenal cortical adenomas are found which are most often non hypersecretory. However, exceptional ACCs have been described in this setting (Libe, 2005).

Diagnosing ACC

Clinical presentation

The clinical features of sporadic ACC are provoked by hormone hypersecretion and/or tumor mass and spread (Luton 1990; Abiven 2003). Other specific features may be associated with rare genetic diseases such as Li-Fraumeni and Wiedemann-Beckwith syndromes, where ACC is part of a more complex syndrome. Rarely, an ACC is diagnosed during the diagnostic work-up for an adrenal incidentaloma (Luton, 2000).

Hypersecretory ACCs

The most common presentation associates features of combined glucocorticoid and androgen oversecretion by the tumor (Luton, 1990; Wajchenberg, 2000; Allolio, 2004; Abiven 2006):

– The first is responsible for Cushing's syndrome: centripetal obesity, protein wasting with skin thinning and striae, muscle atrophy (myopathy), and osteoporosis, impaired defence against infection, diabetes, high blood pressure, psychiatric disturbances, gonadal dysfunction in men and women.

– androgen oversecretion may induce an array of manifestations in women, of increasing severity: hirsutism, menstrual abnormalities, infertility, and eventually franck virilisation (baldness, deepening of the voice, clitoris hypertrophy).

Other biologically active steroids may be oversecreted. Mineralocorticoids, such as DOC (deoxycorticosterone), may contribute a severe state of mineralocorticoid excess with high blood pressure and hypokaliemia. Exceptional tumors with estrogen secretion may provoke gynecomastia in men, metrorragias in post-menopausal women.

A significant subset of ACCs secrete only (or predominantly) a single class of biologically active steroids, androgens most often, but also cortisol in some patients.

Non-hypersecretory ACCs

Some ACCs are "non-hypersecretory" with no clinical features of hormone excess, although they may produce non-bioactive steroid precursors (17OH progesterone).

These latter tumors may be discovered as true "incidentalomas" (Kloos, 1995; Luton 2000), that is, during an imaging procedure that was not related to any adrenal manifestation. Although this situation is not the most frequent, it is increasing, up to 13% in our most recent evaluation of the Cochin cohort of 202 ACCs (Abiven, 2006). We emphasize the crucial importance of correctly diagnosing these tumors, that are most often localized, and thus best candidates for a curative treatment.

More frequently, however, non-hypersecretory ACCs are discovered by the manifestations of the tumor burden: local symptoms (pain, palpation of a tumor), or distant metastases (liver, lung, bones). Fever may occur, concommittant with tumor necrosis. It is quite remarkable, however, that the general state of the patient does not deteriorate in the vast majority of cases even in the presence of an impressive (often metastatic) tumor load. This explains the fact that non hypersecretory ACCs may be diagnosed at a late stage.

Imaging

Imaging is an essential diagnostic step. It analyses the characteristics of the tumor, looking for evidence of malignancy, and contributes to work-up extension and the staging of the tumor (see chapters 4 by Legmann, P. and 8 by Tenenbaum, F.).

Adrenal CT scan is the major tool (Boland 1998): it shows a unilateral mass, that is almost invariably large (above 5-6 cm, often 10 cm and above), lowering the kidney. It shows typical features suggestive of a malignant tumor: the tumor is non homogeneous with foci of necrosis and, sometimes, calcifications; it has irregular margins; its spontaneous density to X-Rays is high (above 20 UH), indicating a low fat content by opposition to what is often found in adenomas. Dynamic measurement of contrast-enhanced densities may provide a more sensitive means to distinguish between benign and malignant lesions. CT also contributes to the detection of local invasion, and distant metastases (liver, lung). Loco-regional vessel invasion through the renal veins and the inferior vena cava can proceed up to the right atrium and result in metastatic lung embolism (Icard 2001).

Adrenal scintigraphy (Gross, 1994) with iodo-cholesterol is not essential, although it can help in special situations.

MRI and/or ultra sound also contribute to the diagnosis of liver nodules, and venous invasions.

Bone scintigraphy may help evaluate bone metastases.

More interestingly, and more recently, studies have demonstrated that ACCs almost always have a high uptake of 18FDG. Thus, 18FDG-Pet scan appears to distinguish between benign and malignant adrenal tumors (Maurea, 2001; Becherer, 2001; Tenenbaum, 2004). This simple, non invasive imaging procedure also contributes to work-up extension (Leboulleux, 2005).

Endocrine Work-up

Routine endocrinological investigations look for oversecretion of various adrenal cortical steroids. When present, they establish the adrenal cortical origin of the tumor.

ACTH-independent cortisol oversecretion is easily detected: increased urinary cortisol excretion, that is not suppressible with high doses of dexamethasone, and associated with undetectable ACTH plasma levels.

Plasma 17OH progresterone is often elevated (baseline and/or after ACTH stimulation), as is the specific adrenal androgen DHEAS which leads to increased plasma testosterone in females. Other steroids such as DOC, Delta 4 androstenedione, and – rarely – estrogens, can be overproduced by the tumor. Exceptional aldosterone producing ACCs have been reported: one should be very careful when faced with such tumors, if they are above 3 cm, with high plasma aldosterone levels, and possibly associated with combined (often subtle) cortisol or other steroid secretion, because they may not be a Conn adenoma!

Again in rare "non-hypersecretory" ACCS, the entire hormonal work-up may be normal.

Evidence for malignancy

At this stage one can accumulate data providing evidence for ACC, and make a first assessment of staging and prognosis, before taking a therapeutic option:

– A large, heterogeneous tumor (above 6 cm), with combined cortisol and androgen hypersecretion leads to an easy diagnosis, with or without evidence of distant metastases.

– A smaller (4-5 cm) tumor with no evidence of steroid secretion, or of local or distant spread, may be a diagnostic problem. The 18FDG Pet scan may be of help when the mass uptakes the tracer (Tenenbaum, 2004).

– Yet, in case of doubt, the presence of a single clue that the lesion might be malignant is an indication for surgery: imaging is not totally reassuring, and/or there is evidence of combined steroid hypersecretion.

A first approach to staging and thus prognosis (see further) can be obtained, through the size of the tumor and the absence or presence of distant metastases.

Surgery

Adrenal tumor

Surgery is key for the treatment since "complete" removal of a localized tumor is the best chance for a cure (Icard, 2001; Schteingart, 2005; Abiven, 2003). It should be performed by an experienced surgeon, with a multidisciplinary team in a referral centre. Whenever there is any doubt that an adrenal tumor may be of malignant origin, the laparoscopic approach should be banned, and a classical laparotomy should be performed. The latter allows the surgeon to perform all the necessary inspection, to remove the tumor and to extend the resection to neighbouring organs in case of local invasion. Thus, open surgery participates in the fine evaluation of the tumor staging. Many ACCs are fragile tumors that must be manipulated with extreme precaution to avoid tumor effraction and tumor cell spilling.

In patients with evidence of glucocorticoid oversecretion, parenteral glucocorticoid aministration is mandatory to prevent adrenal insufficiency after the tumor is removed.

Other surgical approaches

Surgery can also contribute to the treatment of advanced tumors with local invasion and/or distant metastases, either at first operation or after reccurrence (see chapters by Dousset, B and de Baere, T): removal of liver, lung metastases; tumor debulking; threatening bone metastases.

Prognosis

Pathology

Recognizing the malignant nature of an adrenal cortical tumor often remains a challenge even for experienced pathologists (see chapter by Tissier, F). Two sets of criteria have long been used, that are predictors of later tumor reccurrence and/or metastatic spread:

– The tumor size is in itself an excellent predictor of malignancy (Grumbach, 2003): tumors above 6 cm have 25% chance of being malignant; tumors under 4 cm have 2% chance of being malignant. This leaves intermediary tumors (between 4 – 6 cm)...!

– There is not a single pathological feature which allows diagnosis of a malignant adrenal cortical tumor. Pathologists have designed paradigms using a combination of various (independent?) histological parameters that make it possible to establish a "score" for a given tumor. The most widely used is the Weiss score, composed of 9 different items (see chapter by Tissier, F.): each item is given a value of one when it is present, zero when it is absent. The score is obtained by adding the values of each individual item. Since the initial paper by Weiss (1984), it is assumed that a score above 3 is most likely associated with a malignant tumor. We will see further that there is a strong possibility of malignancy at scores of three and even two!

Tumor biology

The limitations of the classical pathological approach have prompted the search for other predictors of malignancy. A number of molecular markers have been shown to be associated with malignant adrenal cortical tumors (see chapter by Bertherat, J.).

Much emphasis has been placed on two gene abnormalities:

– High overexpression of IGF2 is present in an amazingly high number of ACCs (90%), in contrast with adenomas where it is usually normal. More interestingly, it is associated with a specific gene rearrangement at the IGF2 locus leading either to loss of the maternal allele and duplication of the paternal allele, or to loss of the normal maternal imprinting. This gene "turmoil" at 11p15 generates other modification of gene expression that all favour cell growth (Gicquel, 2000; Libe, 2005).
– Loss of allele at the 17p13 locus is also very frequent in ACCs (85%), and almost always absent in adenomas with a Weiss score of 1 or 0. This locus encompasses the *p53* gene. However *p53* mutations are only found in a minority of ACCs, suggesting that a yet unidentified tumor

suppressor gene may be present in this locus. But quite importantly a single prospective study has shown that loss of heterozygosity at 17p13 is an independent predictive factor of malignancy in adrenal cortical tumors (Gicquel, 2001).
– Because these molecular abnormalities (IGF2 mRNA overexpression and/or LOH at 17p13) are already found with high prevalence in tumors with a Weiss score as low as three or two, it is felt that the latter score does not have optimal diagnostic sensitivity *(figure 1)*.
– Recently, overexpression of Cyclin E in the tumor cell was shown to be strongly associated with the malignant phenotype of the tumor (Tissier, 2004). Interestingly, this molecular marker can be assessed using a simple and reproducible technique: immunohistochemistry.

Tumor staging

Several methods of tumor staging have been proposed, that have prognostic implications. The Mc Farlane system (Mc Farlane, 1958) was initially proposed, and remains commonly used:

– Stage 1: local tumor, size less than 5 cm
– Stage 2: local tumor, size more than 5 cm
– Stage 3: any tumor size and mobile nodes or local infiltration reaching neighbouring organs and no lymph node
– Stage 4: any tumor size and invasion of neighbouring organs or fixed nodes or distant metastases

This staging system is best applied after the patient has been operated and distant metastases have been thoroughly searched for, with sensitive means, including 18FDG pet scan.

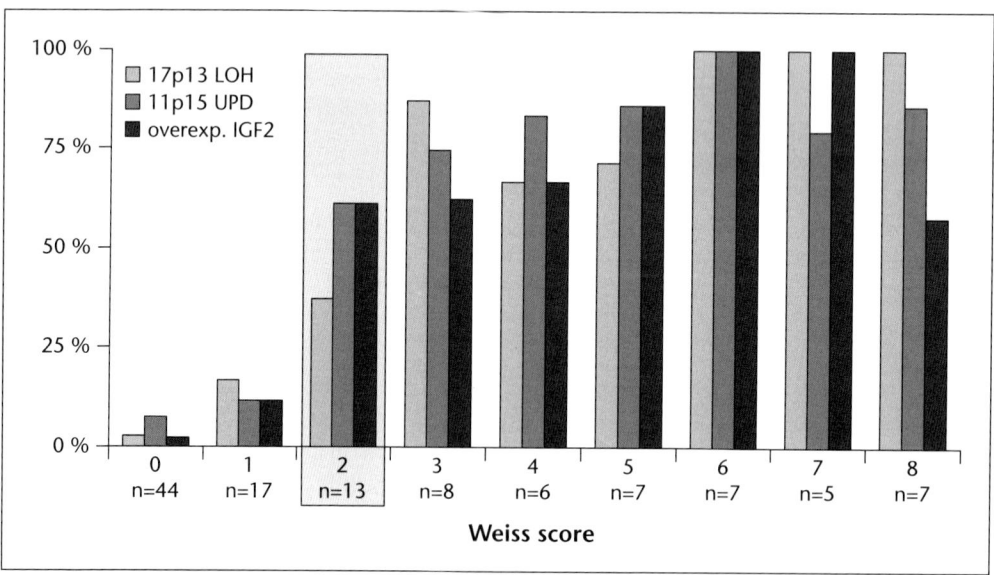

Figure 1. Prevalence of molecular markers of malignancy (IGF2 overexpression, 11p15 LOH, 17p13 LOH), and Weiss score in adrenal cortical tumors. A high prevalence of molecular abnormalities is already present at a Weiss score of 2 (shaded area).

Several studies have convincingly shown that early stage tumors have a better prognosis: in the recent 202 patients cohort of Cochin (Abiven, 2006), the survival rate at five years was 70% for stage 1 tumors, 50% for stage 2 tumors, 10% for stage 3 tumors, 10% for stage 4 tumors *(figure 2)*.

Curative surgery

Curative surgery is obtained when total removal of the tumor (R0) can be performed. This is accomplished in all stage 1 and stage 2 tumors, and in some stage 3 tumors. It requires the surgeon to be experienced in this type of tumor, and a thorough pathological evaluation of the removed tissue. Again, all studies confirm better survival rate after curative surgery (Icard 2001; Schteingart 2005).

Other prognostic factors

In authentic ACCs, numerous other factors predictive of survival have been analyzed. A worse prognosis has been associated with older age at diagnosis, cortisol-hypersecretory tumors, high number of mitoses in the tumor (Medeiros, 1992).

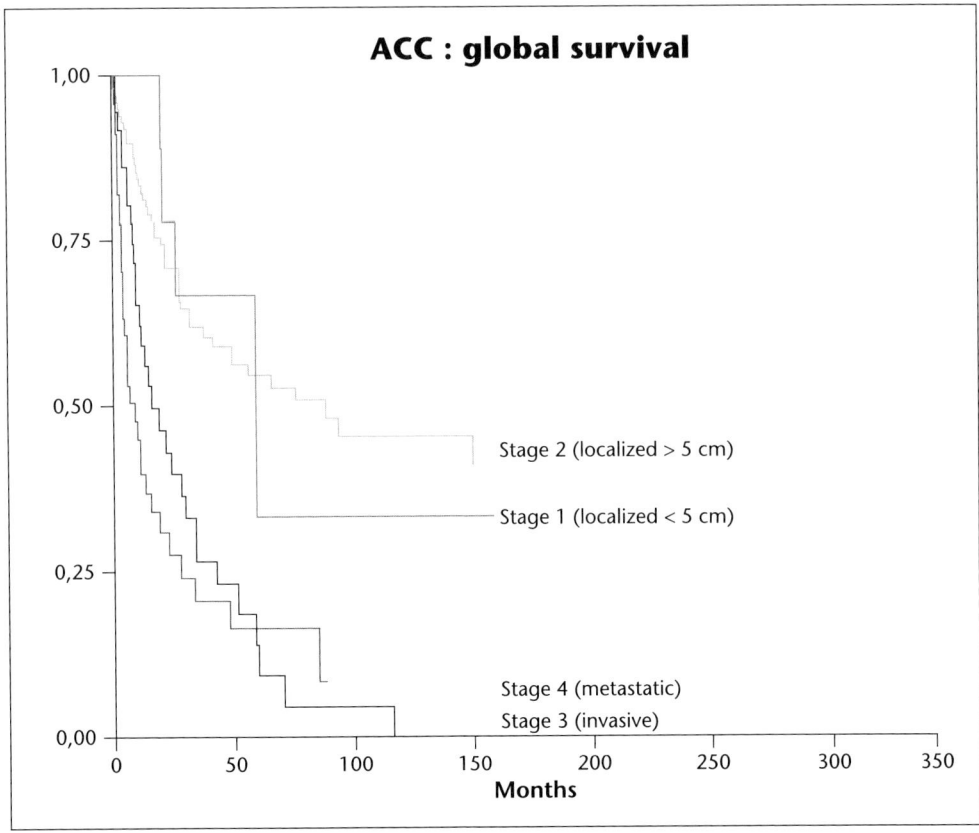

Figure 2. Survival rate according to MacFarlane stage. From Abiven 2006 (with permission).

Chemotherapies

After non-curative surgery, and/or in case of inoperable recurrences or distant metastases, various chemotherapeutic regimens have been used over the years (see chapter 5 by Goldwasser F.).

O, p'DDD (Mitotane, Lysodren®)

O, p'DDD (ortho, para', dichloro-, diphenyl-, dichloro ethane) is a rather specific adrenolytic drug used in various species, including man. It was first used in the mid 1950s in man, and proved to decrease cortisol oversecretion and to exert an antitumoral action in ACCs (Luton, 1990). Retrospective analysis of many studies where the patients were given O, p'DDD shows that total or partial tumor responses were obtained in about 30% of cases, and almost always for only a brief period (Wooten, 1993). In addition, O, p'DDD has numerous side effects (digestive, neurological...) that very often require stopping treatment. Close monitoring of plasma drug concentration is mandatory to ascertain that proper levels are obtained that are high enough to provide a therapeutic effect, and low enough to protect against side effects (van Slooten, 1984; Baudin, 2001). They are available only in specialized centres. Nevertheless, a free plasma testing service is provided to all European centres using Lysodren® (Mitotane, 500 mg)*.

Although far from ideal, O, p'DDD is considered by most authors as a reference treatment.

Yet in most patients a beneficial effect with O, p'DDD either is not observed or is transient.

Other chemotherapies

Many other chemotherapeutic regimens have been tested over the years. Because ACC is a rare disease, only small groups of patients have been studied, and no controlled (randomized) approach has ever been used.

Among the various tentative treatments that can be analyzed through the literature (Allolio, 2004), two have shown a possible benefit: combined treatment with Cis-platine, Etoposide, Doxorubicin, given with O, p'DDD (Berruti, 2005), and Streptozotocin given with O, p'DDD (Khan, 2000), with response rates (complete or partial tumor regression) of 48% and 36% respectively.

These are, of course, unacceptable response rates, and it is fair to say that no fully efficacious medical treatment for ACC is known to date.

Other therapeutic means

External radiotherapy for the prevention or treatment of local recurrence has occasionally been reported to have some success. Yet it is not generally accepted that ACCs are radiosensitive. In contrast, external radiotherapy can prove highly efficient in the treatment of bone metastases.

---

* www.lysodren-europe.com

Chemoembolisation, and/or radiofrequeny ablation may also be used to treat local recurrences, and/or metastases, particularly in the liver, lung, and bones (see chapter by de Baere, T.).

Strategy *(figure 3)*

The first step is to recognize the likelihood that an adrenal tumor might be an ACC. This helps to avoid laparoscopic surgery and the risk of tumor cell seeding along the extractive pathway of the tumor. It indicates that a thorough staging work-up be performed, that the patient be operated by an experienced surgeon, and the tumor be analyzed as well by an experienced pathologist.

After "curative" surgery in stage 1 and 2 tumors, and in some stage 3 tumors, close surveillance is mandatory since recurrence will eventually occur in more than half the patients. It is questionable whether adjuvant chemotherapy with O, p' DDD limits the rate of recurrence and increases survival.

In stage 3 and 4 tumors, when "curative" surgery is impossible, and at the time of local recurrence and/or metastases spread after "curative" surgery, the following gross principle can be followed:

– Second surgery, when all the tumor can be removed (local recurrence, isolated liver or lung metastases).

– Tumor debulking may help abrogate loco-regional complications and/or steroid oversecretion. Chemoembolisation or radiofrequency ablation may be of help.

– Systemic chemotherapy is mandatory, generally with O,p'DDD as a first line treatment. After O,p'DDD has failed, other chemotherapeutic regimens are discussed.

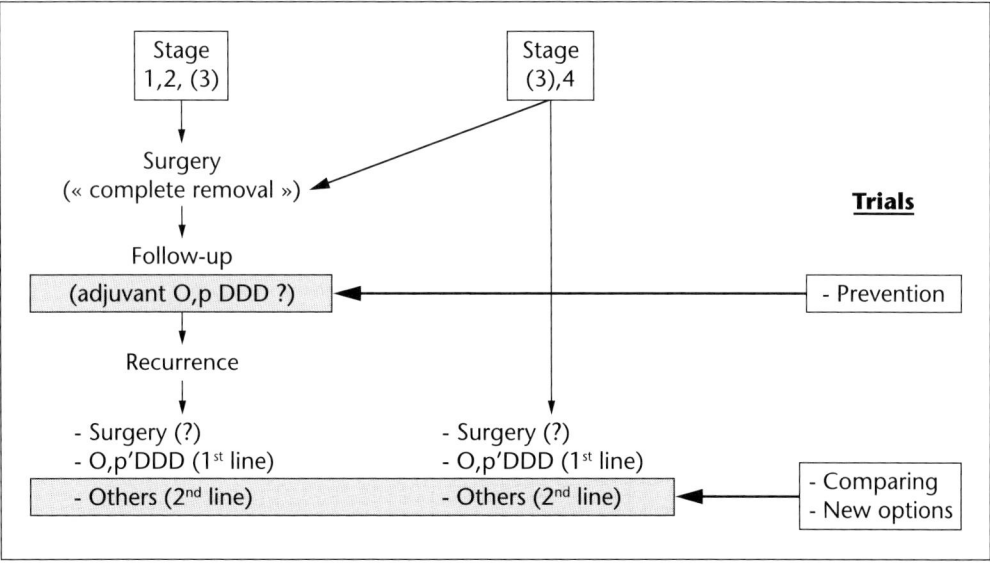

Figure 3. Treatment strategy for ACC.

Perspectives *(figure 4)*

Transcriptome analysis of adrenocortical tumors has already provided us with encouraging data that help distinguish benign from malignant tumors (Giordano, 2003; de Fraipont, 2005). Further studies (in progress) should eventually allow much better insight into the fine biology of each individual tumor, and its particular prognosis.

The fine pathophysiological mechanisms of tumorigenesis in adrenocortical tumors are being more and more recognized. The roles of the IGF-2/IGF-type 1 receptor pathway, of the wnt/β-catenin pathway (Tissier, 2005), of the 11p15 locus, of angiogenic pathways, have been well recognized for many years or more recently identified. They point to new molecular actors that will, hopefully, become new molecular targets for future therapeutic methods.

Because ACC is a rare disease, it is necessary that research and clinical management of patients be organized in national and international networks. These networks (COMETE in France, GANIMED in Germany, NISGAT in Italy, and ENS@T in Europe) make it possible to provide the most sophisticated investigative tools to all patients, and they are crucial for launching therapeutic trials (Kirschner, 2006) with a sufficient number of patients (see the FIRM-ACT trial in the chapter by Goldwasser F.).

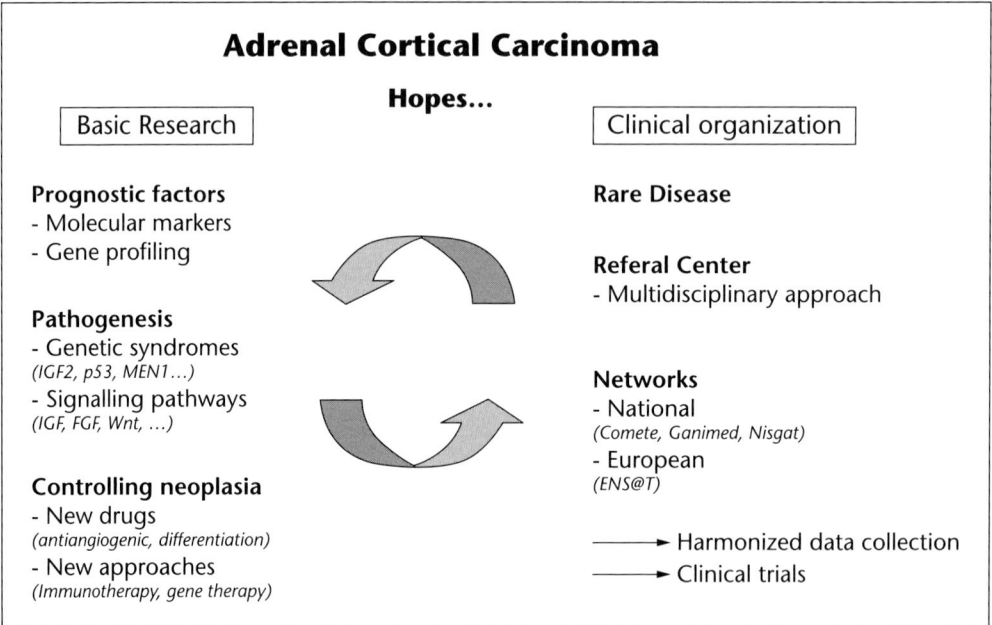

Figure 4. Hopes... and perspectives in ACC.

References

Abiven G, Coste J, Groussin L, et al. Clinical and biological features in the prognosis of adrenal cortical carcinoma. Poor outcome of cortisol secreting tumors in a series of 202 consecutive patients. *J Clin Endocrinol Metab* 2006; 91: 2650-55.

Allolio B, Hahner S, Weismann D, Fassnacht M. Management of adrenocortical carcinoma. *Clin Endocrinol* (Oxf) 2004; 60 (3): 273-87. Review.

Baudin E, Pellegriti G, Bonnay M, et al. Impact of monitoring plasma 1, 1-dichlorodiphenildichloroethane (O,p'DDD) levels on the treatment of patients with adrenocortical carcinoma. *Cancer* 2001; 92 (6): 1385-92.

Becherer A, Vierhapper H, Potzi C, et al. FDG-PET in adrenocortical carcinoma. *Cancer Biother Radiopharm* 2001; 16 (4): 289-95.

Berruti A, Terzolo M, Sperone P, et al. Etoposide, doxorubicin and cisplatin plus mitotane in the treatment of advanced adrenocortical carcinoma: a large prospective phase II trial. *Endocr Relat Cancer* 2005; 12 (3): 657-66.

Boland GW, Lee MJ, Gazelle GS, Halpern EF, McNicholas MM, Mueller PR. Characterization of adrenal masses using unenhanced CT: an analysis of the CT. literature. *Am J Roentgenol* 1998; 171 (1): 201-4.

De Fraipont F, El Atifi M, Cherradi N, Le Moigne G, Defaye G, Houlgatte R, Bertherat J, Bertagna X, Plouin PF, Baudin E, Berger F, Gicquel C, Chabre O, Feige JJ. Gene expression profiling of human adrenocortical tumors using complementary deoxyribonucleic Acid microarrays identifies several candidate genes as markers of malignancy. *J Clin Endocrinol Metab* 2005; 90 (3): 1819-29.

Gicquel C, Bertherat J, Le Bouc Y, Bertagna X. Pathogenesis of adrenocortical incidentalomas and genetic syndromes associated with adrenocortical neoplasms. *Endocrinol Metab Clin North Am* 2000; 29 (1): 1-13, vii. Review.

Gicquel C, Bertagna X, Gaston V, Coste J, Louvel A, Baudin E, Bertherat J, Chapuis Y, Duclos JM, Schlumberger M, Plouin PF, Luton JP, Le Bouc Y. Molecular markers and long-term recurrences in a large cohort of patients with sporadic adrenocortical tumors. *Cancer Res* 2001; 61 (18): 6762-7.

Giordano TJ, Thomas DG, Kuick R, Lizynes M, Misek DE, Smith AL, Sanders D, Aljundi RT, Gauger PG, Thompson NW, Taylor JM, Hanash SM. Distinct transcriptional profiles of adrenocortical tumors uncovered by DNA microarray analysis. *Am J Pathol* 2003; 162 (2): 521-31.

Gross MG, Shapiro B, Francis IR. Scintigraphic evaluation of clinically silent adrenal masses. *J Nucl Med* 1994; 35: 1145-52.

Grumbach MM, Biller BM, Braunstein GD, Campbell KK, Carney JA, Godley PA, Harris EL, Lee JK, Oertel YC, Posner MC, Schlechte JA, Wieand HS. Management of the clinically inapparent adrenal mass ("incidentaloma"). *Ann Intern Med* 2003; 138 (5): 424-9.

Icard P, Goudet P, Charpenay C, Andreassian B, Carnaille B, Chapuis Y, Cougard P, Henry JF, Proye C. Adrenocortical carcinomas: surgical trends and results of a 253-patient series from the French Association of Endocrine Surgeons study group. *World J Surg* 2001; 25 (7): 891-7.

Khan TS, Imam H, Juhlin C, Skogseid B, Grondal S, Tibblin S, Wilander E, Oberg K, Eriksson B. Streptozocin and o, p'DDD in the treatment of adrenal cortical carcinoma patients: long-term survival in its adjuvant use. *Ann Oncol* 2000; 11 (10): 1281-7.

Kirschner LS. Emerging treatment strategies for adrenocortical carcinoma: a new hope. *J Clin Endocrinol Metab* 2006; 91 (1): 14-21. *Epub* 2005. Review.

Kloos RT, Gross RT, Francis IR, Korobkin M, Shapiro B. Incidentally discovered adrenal masses. *Endocrine Rev* 1995; 16: 460-84.

Leboulleux S, Dromain C, Bonniaud G, Auperin A, Caillou B, Lumbroso J, Sigal R, Baudin E, Schlumberger M. Diagnostic and prognostic value of 18-fluorodeoxyglucose positron emission tomography in adrenocortical carcinoma: a prospective comparison with computed tomography. *J Clin Endocrinol Metab* 2005; 91: 920-5.

Libe R, Bertherat J. Molecular genetics of adrenocortical tumors, from familial to sporadic diseases. *Eur J Endocrinol* 2005; 153 (4): 477-87. Review.

Luton JP, Cerdas S, Billaud L, Thomas G, Guilhaume B, Bertagna X, Laudat MH, Louvel A, Chapuis Y, Blondeau P, et al. Clinical features of adrenocortical carcinoma, prognostic factors, and the effect of mitotane therapy. *N Engl J Med* 1990; 322 (17): 1195-201.

Luton JP, Martinez M, Coste J, Bertherat J. Outcome in patients with adrenal incidentaloma selected for surgery: an analysis of 88 cases investigated in a single clinical center. *Eur J Endocrinol* 2000; 143 (1): 111-7.

Mac Farlane DA. Cancer of the adrenal cortex: the natural history, prognosis and treatment in the study of 58 cases. *Ann Royal Coll Surg* 1958; 109: 613-8.

Medeiros LJ, Weiss LM. New developments in the pathologic diagnosis of adrenal cortical neoplasms. A review. *Am J Clin Pathol* 1992; 97 (1): 73-83. Review.

Schteingart DE, Doherty GM, Gauger PG, Giordano TJ, Hammer GD, Korobkin M, Worden FP. Management of patients with adrenal cancer: recommendations of an international consensus conference. *Endocr Relat Cancer* 2005; 12 (3): 667-80. Review.

Tenenbaum F, Groussin L, Foehrenbach H, Tissier F, Gouya H, Bertherat J, Dousset B, Legmann P, Richard B, Bertagna X. 18F-fluorodeoxyglucose positron emission tomography as a diagnostic tool for malignancy of adrenocortical tumors? Preliminary results in 13 consecutive patients. *Eur J Endocrinol* 2004; 150 (6): 789-92.

Tissier F, Louvel A, Grabar S, Hagnere AM, Bertherat J, Vacher-Lavenu MC, Dousset B, Chapuis Y, Bertagna X, Gicquel C. Cyclin E correlates with malignancy and adverse prognosis in adrenocortical tumors. *Eur J Endocrinol* 2004; 150 (6): 809-17.

Tissier F, Cavard C, Groussin L, Perlemoine K, Fumey G, Hagnere AM, Renc-Corail F, Jullian E, Gicquel C, Bertagna X, Vacher-Lavenu MC, Perret C, Bertherat J. Mutations of beta-catenin in adrenocortical tumors: activation of the Wnt signaling pathway is a frequent event in both benign and malignant adrenocortical tumors. *Cancer Res* 2005; 65 (17): 7622-7.

Van Slooten H, Moolenaar AJ, van Seters AP, Smeenk D. The treatment of adrenocortical carcinoma with o, p'-DDD: prognostic implications of serum level monitoring. *Eur J Cancer Clin Oncol* 1984; 20 (1): 47-53.

Wajchenberg BL, Albergaria-Pereira MA, Medonca BB, Latronico AC, Campo-Carneiro P, Alves VA, Zerbini MC, Liberman B, Carlos-Gomes G, Kirschner MA. Adrenocortical carcinoma: clinical and laboratory observations. *Cancer* 2000; 88 (4): 711-36. Review.

Weiss LM. Comparative histologic study of 43 metastasizing and nonmetastasizing adrenocortical tumors. *Am J Surg Pathol* 1984; 8 (3): 163-9.

Wooten MD, King DK. Adrenal cortical carcinoma. Epidemiology and treatment with mitotane and a review of the literature. *Cancer* 1993; 72 (11): 3145-55.

Molecular genetics of adrenal cortical carcinoma

Rossella Libé[1], Christine Gicquel[2], Xavier Bertagna[1,3], Jérôme Bertherat[1,3]
1. INSERM U567 and CNRS UMR 8104, Institut Cochin, Paris
2. Functional Investigation Department, A. Trousseau Hospital, Paris
3. Endocrine and Metabolic Diseases, Cochin Hospital, APHP, Univ. Paris 5

Progress in the understanding of the pathogenesis and molecular genetics of adrenal cortical carcinoma (ACC) has been slower than for other tumors. This can be easily explained by the rarity of these malignant neoplasms. However, considerable advances toward understanding the molecular mechanisms of adrenal cortical tumor (ACT) development have been made in the last decade. Several observations have demonstrated that genetic alterations are frequent in both benign and especially in malignant ACTs. The study of rare genetic syndromes associated with ACC has greatly facilitated this progress, and has increased our understanding of the mechanisms of ACC development.

Chromosomal alterations and clonal origin of adrenal cortical carcinomas

The study of tumor clonality is important to establish the cellular origins of neoplasms and to identify the mechanisms underlying tumor progression. Polyclonality suggests that tumor cells are affected by local or systemic stimuli, whereas monoclonality indicates that tumor progression is the end result of an intrinsic genetic mutation. In two different studies, analysis of the pattern of X-chromosome inactivation in heterozygous female tissues has shown that ACCs consist of monoclonal populations of cells and that nodular hyperplastic adrenal tissue consists of a polyclonal population of cells (Beuschlein, 1994; Gicquel, 1994b).

Once a subclone acquires a genetic advantage over competing subclones, selective proliferation may occur, with the advantaged clone replacing other cells in the tumor. This suggests that a first genetic event might be present in ACC development, leading to proliferation of a monoclonal cell population. Several of these genetic alterations have been identified since these original studies on the clonality of ACC.

These genetic events can be studied at the scale of the whole genome, as losses or gains of part or all of a chromosome. A large number of molecular techniques, such as comparative genomic hybridisation (CGH) and microsatellite analysis can be used in genome-wide screening for such chromosomal alterations. These approaches have identified alterations affecting various chromosomes and loci. Interestingly, a correlation has been observed between tumor size and the number of CGH changes in ACT, suggesting that chromosomal alterations could accumulate during ACT progression (Sidhu, 2002) *(figure 1)*. It was demonstrated by CGH that chromosomal alterations are observed in 28% of benign ACTs (Kjellman, 1996). Most of the changes observed concern losses on chromosomes 2, 11q and 17p and gains on chromosomes 4 and 5 (Dohna, 2000; Kjellman, 1999; Sidhu, 2002; Zhao, 1999). In more recent studies, CGH identified changes in 61% of benign ACTs, and the most common gains observed were on chromosomes 5, 12, 19 and 4 (Sidhu, 2002). Losses were observed at 1p, 17p, 22p, 22q, 2q and 11q in up to 62% of cases of ACC. Studies using microsatellite markers have demonstrated a high percentage of loss of heterozygosity/allelic imbalance (LOH/AI) at 11q13 (100%) and 2p16 (92%) in carcinomas (Kjellman, 1999). Moreover, LOH of the 17p13 locus has been reported to be more frequent in malignant tumors and to be of prognostic value for the recurrence of localized tumors (Gicquel, 2001).

From germline to somatic genetic alterations in adrenal cortical carcinoma *(table I)*

Li-Fraumeni, TP53 and the 17p13 locus

TP53 is a tumor suppressor gene, located at 17p13, and involved in the control of cell proliferation. Acquired mutations in *TP53* are common tumor-specific genetic alterations in humans, and have been identified in various cancers. Germline mutations in *TP53* are identified in 70% of families with Li-Fraumeni Syndrome (LFS). This syndrome displays dominant inheritance and confers susceptibility to breast carcinoma, soft tissue sarcoma, brain tumors, osteosarcoma, leukaemia and ACC (Hisada, 1998). These tumors have an early onset, affecting mostly children and young adults. Germline mutations in *TP53* have been observed in 50-80% of children with apparently sporadic ACC in North America and Europe (Varley, 1999). The incidence of pediatric ACC is about 10 times higher in Southern Brazil than in the rest of the world, and a specific germline mutation has been identified in exon 10 of the *TP53* gene (R337H) in almost all cases (Latronico, 2001; Ribeiro, 2001). Molecular studies about this mutation have shown that the tissue-specific effects of this mutation may be due to a pH-dependent effect caused by the replacement of an arginine by a histidine in the tetramerisation domain of TP53 (DiGiammarino, 2002).

In sporadic ACC in adults, somatic mutations of *TP53* are found in only 25% of ACC cases and are located in four "hot spot regions" within exons 5 and 8, as first demonstrated (Ohgaki, 1993; Reincke, 1994). A more recent study suggests a *TP53* mutation rate of 70% in ACC (Barzon, 2001).

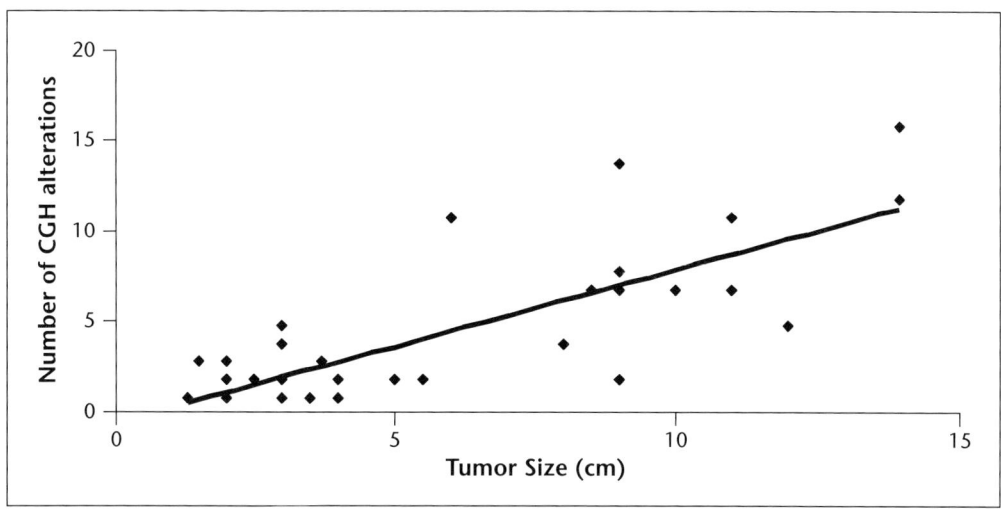

Figure 1. Correlation between tumor size and the number of chromosomal alterations studied by Comparative Genomic Hybridization in adrenal cortical tumors.
The figure shows the significant correlation between tumor size and the number of CGH alterations in ACT (adapted from the work of S. Sidhu *et al.*, 2002). ACC are usually among the largest (> 5 cm) tumors, and tumors below 3 cm are usually benign tumors.

Loss of heterozygosity (LOH) at 17p13 has been consistently demonstrated in ACC (reviewed in Libe & Bertherat, 2005). LOH at 17p13 occurs in 85% of ACC and is extremely rare in benign adrenocortical adenomas (Gicquel, 2001) *(figure 2)*. LOH at 17p13 is correlated with Weiss score – an index of cytopathological alterations used to determine the malignancy of ACT. It has therefore been suggested that 17p13 LOH could be used as a molecular marker of malignancy in ACT (see chapter by Bertagna X.). In a large prospective study of ACT patients, 17p13 LOH was also demonstrated to be an independent variable predictive of recurrence after complete surgical removal of localised ACT (Gicquel, 2001) *(figure 3)*.

The discrepancy between the frequencies of *TP53* mutation and 17p13 LOH may be accounted for by the existence of another tumor suppressor gene in this region. The *HIC-1* gene (hypermethylated in cancer) is a possible candidate. It encodes a transcription factor triggered by TP53 and inactivated by hypermethylation or allelic losses in various cancers.

Multiple Endocrine Neoplasia type 1, the menin gene and the 11q13 locus

The *menin* gene, located at the 11q13 locus, is a tumor suppressor gene. A heterozygous inactivating germline mutation of *menin* is found in about 90% of families affected by multiple endocrine neoplasia type 1 (MEN 1). This is an autosomal dominant syndrome with high penetrance. The principal clinical features include parathyroid (95%), endocrine pancreas (45%) and pituitary (45%) tumors. Adrenocortical tumors and/or hyperplasia are observed in 25-40% of MEN 1 patients (Kjellman, 1999; Schulte, 2000). In most cases, they are non-hypersecreting

Table I. Summary of the genetic syndromes associated with ACC.

Gene and chromosomal localisation	Genetic disease	Tumors and associated manifestations	Sporadic ACC
TP53 (17p13) (hCHK2)	Li-Fraumeni syndrome (LFS)	Soft tissue sarcoma, breast cancers, brain tumors, leukaemia, ACC	– TP53 germline mutation in paediatric ACC – TP53 somatic mutations in sporadic ACC – 17p13 LOH in sporadic ACC
Menin (11q13)	Multiple endocrine neoplasia type 1 (MEN 1)	Parathyroid, pituitary, pancreas tumors Adrenal cortex: adenoma, hyperplasia, rare carcinoma	– Very rare menin gene mutations in sporadic adrenocortical tumors – Frequent 11q13 LOH in ACC
CDKN1C (p57kip2) mutation KCNQ1OT1 (epigenetic defect) H19 (epigenetic defect) 11p15 locus alterations IGF-II overexpression	Beckwith-Wiedemann syndrome (BWS)	Omphalocele, macroglossia, macrosomia, hemihypertrophy, Wilms' tumor, ACT	– 11p15 paternal isodisomy in ACC – IGF-II overexpression in ACC
APC (5q12-22)	Familial Adenomatous Polyposis (FAP)	Multiple adenomatous polyps and cancer of the colon and rectum. Possible extracolonic manifestations: periampullary cancer, thyroid tumors, hepatoblastoma, rare cases of ACC, ACA, multiples or bilateral ACA Congenital hypertrophy of the retinal pigment epithelium (CHRPE)	– Transcriptome analysis shows Wnt-signaling activation in ACC – β-catenin somatic mutations in ACT

This table describes genetic diseases responsible for adrenocortical tumors (that could be often, or in rare cases, malignant) and other tumoral and non-tumoral manifestations. The molecular alterations in the genes responsible observed in sporadic adrenocortical tumors (mostly at the somatic level) are listed in the "sporadic tumors" column. ACA: adrenocortical adenoma. ACC: adrenal cortical carcinoma. ACT: adrenocortical tumor. LOH: allelic loss

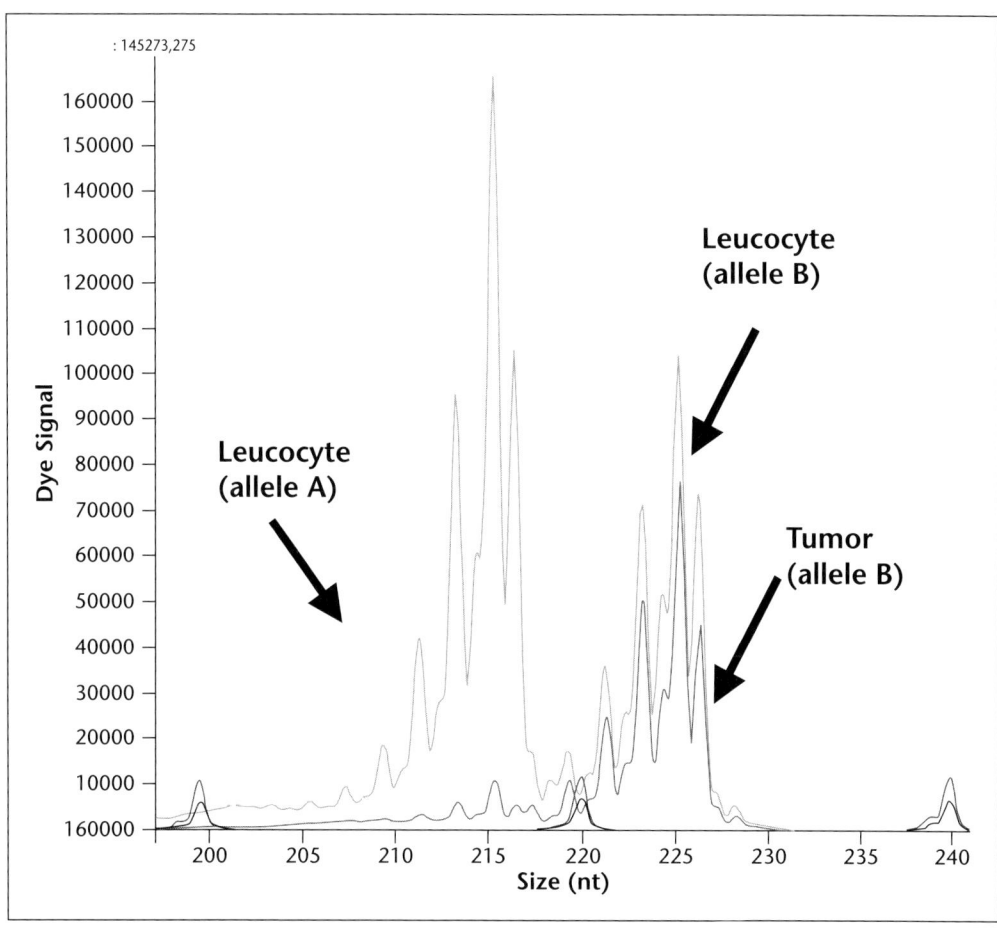

Figure 2. Loss of heterozygosity (LOH) at 17p13 in adrenal cortical carcinoma.
The figure shows the result of LOH study by microsatelitte analysis in an ACC. Briefly, patient leucocyte and tumor DNA are amplified by PCR using fluorescent primers. The PCR products are analyzed on an automated sequencer. The microsatellite marker shown here is informative since two different alleles, A and B, are observed at the level of the leucocyte (germline) DNA. But contrast analysis of the tumor DNA shows only one allele (allele B), demonstrating that LOH occurs at this locus in this ACC.

adrenocortical adenomas that can be managed conservatively with radiological/hormonal follow-up. Hyperplasia is typically also found in MEN 1 patients presenting with ACTH hypersecretion (Cushing's disease), whereas ACC has been observed in rare cases of MEN 1 patients.

Somatic mutation of the *MEN1* gene in sporadic ACT is very rare: one mutation was identified in a series of 41 adrenocortical adenomas in one study, and one mutation in a series of ACC was found in another (Heppner, 1999; Schulte, 2000). By contrast, LOH at 11q13 was identified in more than 90% of informative ACC in three different series, whereas it has been

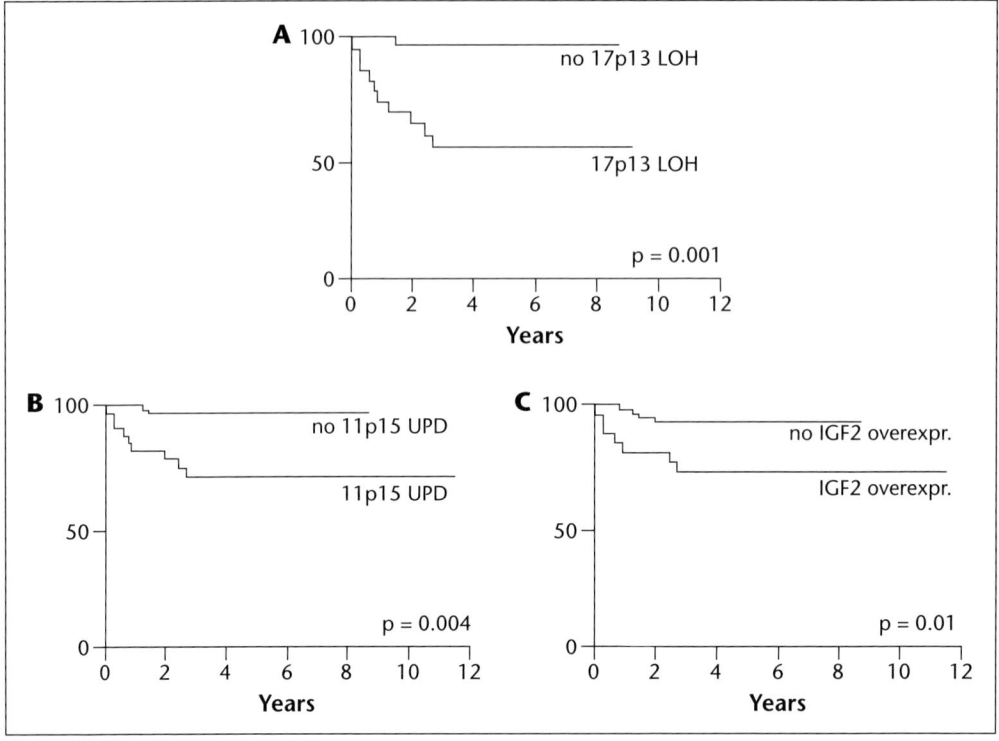

Figure 3. Molecular alterations and adrenocortical tumor recurrence.
The figure shows Kaplan-Meier disease free survival analysis in 96 patients with localized adrenocortical tumors completely removed by surgery (from C. Gicquel et al., 2001) according to 17p13 LOH (panel A), 11p15 paternal isodisomy (panel B) and IGF-II overexpression (panel C). The disease free survival is significantly shorter when one of these molecular alterations is present.

reported in less than 20% of informative adenomas. However, LOH in ACC involves almost all of the 11q domain, suggesting that an as yet unidentified tumor suppressor gene located on the long arm of chromosome 11 may be involved in ACC formation.

Beckwith-Wiedemann, IGF-II (insulin-like growth factor II) and 11p15 alterations *(figure 4)*

The 11p15 region is organized into two different clusters: a telomeric domain including the *IGF-II* and H19 genes and a centromeric domain including the *CDKN1C (p57kip2), KCNQ1OT1* and *KCNQ1* genes. The *IGF-II* gene encodes an important foetal growth factor, is maternally imprinted and is therefore expressed only from the paternal allele (Gicquel, 2000). The *H19* mRNA is not translated and this gene may modulate *IGF-II* expression. The CDKN1C *(p57kip2)* gene encodes a cyclin-dependent kinase inhibitor involved in the G1/S phase of the cell cycle. The *H19* and CDKN1C genes are paternally imprinted and are therefore expressed from the maternal allele only.

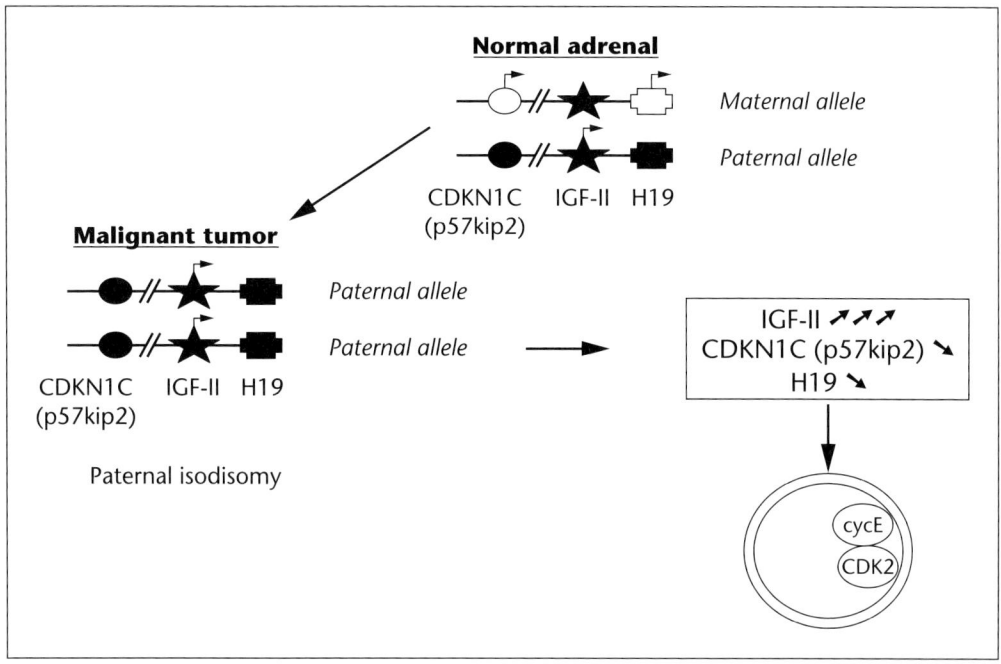

Figure 4. Schematic representation of changes at the 11p15 locus in adrenal cortical carcinomas. The imprinted 11p15 locus contains the *CDKN1C (p57kip2)*, *IGF-II* and *H19* genes. In normal differentiated tissue, only the paternal allele of the *IGF-II* gene is expressed, whereas here only the maternal alleles of *CDKN1C* and *H19* are expressed. Paternal isodisomy is usually observed in adrenal cancers with allelic losses at 11p15. This leads to overexpression of *IGF-II* and decreases the expression of *CDKN1C* and *H19*. This, in turn, affects the cell cycle, leading to overproduction of cyclin E and CDK2 (from reference (Libe et al., 2005), with permission).

Genetic or epigenetic changes of one or of the two imprinted domains of the 11p15 region resulting in an increase in *IGF-II* expression have been implicated in Beckwith-Wiedemann syndrome (BWS) (reviewed in Gaston et al., 2001). This overgrowth disorder is characterised by macrosomia, macroglossia, organomegaly and developmental abnormalities (in particular abdominal wall defects with ex-omphalos). It predisposes patients to the development of embryonal tumors – such as Wilms' tumor, ACT, neuroblastoma and hepatoblastoma.

The insulin-like growth factors system is involved in the development and maintenance of differentiated adrenocortical functions and its role has been largely documented in ACT (Gicquel, 1994a).

Many studies have demonstrated that *IGF-II* is strongly overexpressed in malignant adrenocortical tumors, with overexpression observed in approximately 90% of ACC (Gicquel, 2001). Transcriptome analysis of ACT has demonstrated that *IGF-II* is the most overexpressed gene in ACC by comparison with adrenocortical adenomas or normal adrenal glands (de Fraipont, 2005; Giordano, 2003). The mechanism underlying *IGF-II* overexpression is paternal isodisomy (loss of the maternal allele and duplication of the paternal allele) or, less frequently, loss of imprinting (with maintenance of both parental alleles but a paternal-like *IGF-II* gene expression pattern) (Gicquel, 2000).

Receptors for IGF-I and IGF-II are present in adrenal tissues and strong overexpression of intact IGF-I receptors has been shown in ACC (Weber, 1997). The mitogenic effect of *IGF-II* is dependent on the IGF-I receptor (Logie, 1999). IGF-II is involved in the ACC NCI H295R cell line proliferation and ACTs *via* the IGF-I receptor. IGF-II effects are restricted to tumors, and plasma IGF-II concentrations are usually in the normal range. The biological effects of IGFs are modulated *in vivo* by six IGF-binding proteins (IGFBPs), which positively or negatively regulate the effects of IGFs, depending on their abundance and affinity for growth factors. H295R cells and adrenocortical tumors with IGF-II overproduction have been shown to contain large amounts of IGFBP-2 (Boulle, 1998), suggesting that IGFBP-2 may regulate IGF-II effects in ACC.

In normal adrenocortical tissue, only the maternal *H19* allele is expressed and expression of this gene is abolished in most ACCs displaying paternal isodisomy (Gicquel, 1997). Expression of *CDKN1C* is also abolished in ACC (Liu, 1997). Like 17p13 LOH, 11p15 paternal isodisomy is associated with a higher risk of tumor recurrence, is more frequent in ACC than in adrenocortical adenomas (78.5 *vs* 9.5%) and correlates with the Weiss score (Gicquel, 2001). Thus, 11p15 alterations could be used as a biological marker for predicting ACC malignancy after surgical removal of the tumor. However, 11p15 paternal isodisomy seems to have a lower predictive value than 17p13 LOH (Gicquel, 2001).

The WNT-signalling pathway in adrenocortical tumors

Genetic alterations of the Wnt signalling pathway was initially identified in familial adenomatous polyposis coli and have been extended to a variety of cancers (Kikuchi, 2003). Adrenocortical tumors have been reported in some case reports of patients with FAP (Naylor, 1981). Furthermore, FAP patients with germ-line mutations of the *APC* (Adenomatous Polyposis Coli) gene that lead to an activation of the Wnt signaling pathway may develop ACTs (Blaker, 2004). Molecular studies have suggested that somatic mutations of APC could occur in these tumors in patients already having a germ-line defect.

The Wnt signaling pathway is normally activated during embryonic development. β-catenin is a key component of this signaling pathway. It has a structural role in cell-cell adhesion, and is a transcription cofactor with T cell factor/lymphoid enhancer factor (TCF/LEF) mediating transcriptional activation of target genes of the Wnt signaling pathway *(figure 5)*.

Interestingly, gene profiling studies in various types of ACT have shown the frequent activation of Wnt signaling target genes: in ACC a microarray approach has shown that Ectodermal-Neural Cortex one (ECN-1) was up-regulated (Giordano, 2003). In both benign and malignant ACT, β-catenin accumulation can be observed. These alterations seem very frequent in ACC,

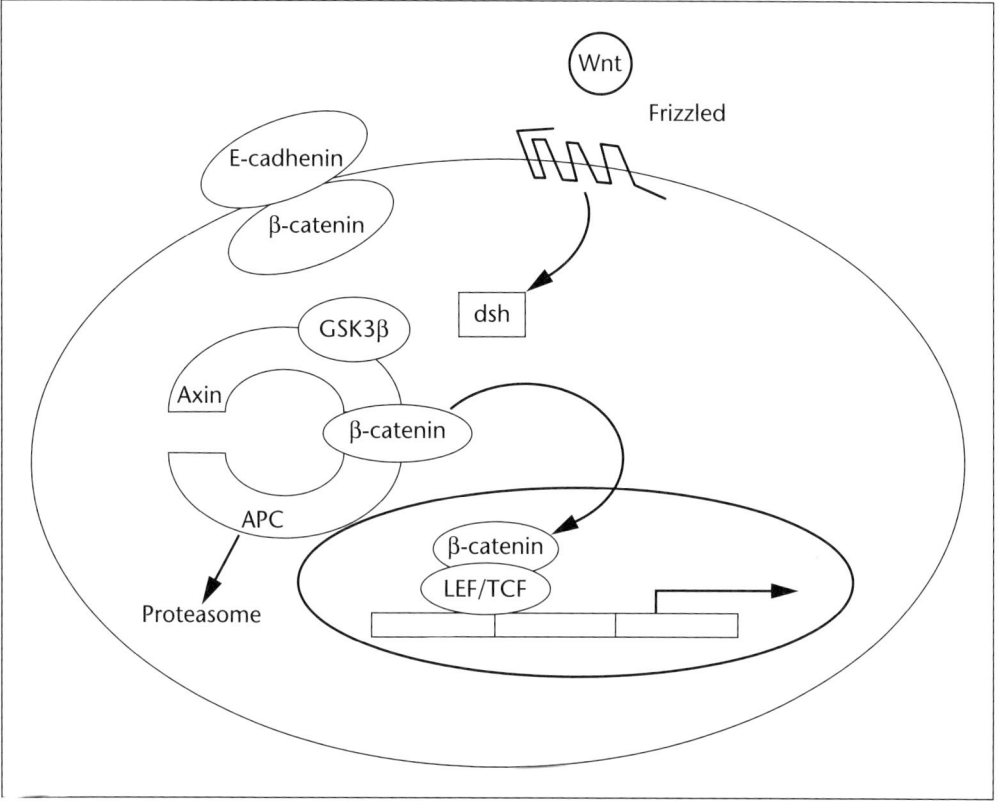

Figure 5. The Wnt signalling pathway.
In the absence of Wnt signalling, the level of β-catenin is low due to degradation by the ubiquitin-proteasome system after phosphorylation by the GSK3-β kinase bound to a scaffolding complex of axin and APC. Wnt stimulation leads to the inactivation of GSK3-β and thereby the stabilization of β-catenin in the cytoplasm. After translocation in the nucleus, β-catenin stimulates target gene expression after interaction with LEF/TCF (T cell factor/lymphoid enhancer factor).

consistent with an abnormal activation of the Wnt-signaling pathway. This is explained in a subset of ACT by somatic mutations of the β-catenin gene altering the GSK3-β phosphorylation site (Tissier, 2005).

Conclusion

Studies of clonality and gene rearrangement in ACT clearly show that genetic alterations play a major role in adrenal cortex tumorigenesis. Studies of hereditary neoplasia syndromes have led to the identification of various loci or chromosomal regions and genes responsible for ACC development. The same molecular defects are observed in the germline DNA in cases of hereditary disease and in somatic DNA in cases of sporadic ACT. For a given genetic defect, the tumor phenotype observed in sporadic tumors displays some similarities to the tumor phenotype observed in familial diseases. This may have important clinical implications as the molecular study of tumor DNA could provide important information for diagnostic and/or prognostic purposes. In the future, targeted therapy might be developed for ACC from the understanding of these key genetic defects that are important for tumor development and progression.

References

Barzon L, Chilosi M, Fallo F, et al. Molecular analysis of CDKN1C and TP53 in sporadic adrenal tumors. *Eur J Endocrinol* 2001; 145 (2): 207-12.

Beuschlein F, Reincke M, Karl M, et al. Clonal composition of human adrenocortical neoplasms. *Cancer Res* 1994; 54 (18): 4927-32.

Blaker H, Sutter C, Kadmon M, et al. Analysis of somatic APC mutations in rare extracolonic tumors of patients with familial adenomatous polyposis coli. *Genes Chromosomes Cancer* 2004; 41 (2): 93-8.

Boulle N, Logie A, Gicquel C, Perin L, Le Bouc Y. Increased levels of insulin-like growth factor II (IGF-II) and IGF-binding protein-2 are associated with malignancy in sporadic adrenocortical tumors. *J Clin Endocrinol Metab* 1998; 83 (5): 1713-20.

de Fraipont F, El Atifi M, Cherradi N, et al. Gene expression profiling of human adrenocortical tumors using complementary deoxyribonucleic Acid microarrays identifies several candidate genes as markers of malignancy. *J Clin Endocrinol Metab* 2005; 90 (3): 1819-29.

DiGiammarino EL, Lee AS, Cadwell C, et al. A novel mechanism of tumorigenesis involving pH-dependent destabilization of a mutant p53 tetramer. *Nat Struct Biol* 2002; 9 (1): 12-6.

Dohna M, Reincke M, Mincheva A, Allolio B, Solinas-Toldo S, Lichter P. Adrenocortical carcinoma is characterized by a high frequency of chromosomal gains and high-level amplifications. *Genes Chromosomes Cancer* 2000; 28 (2): 145-52.

Gaston V, Le Bouc Y, Soupre V, et al. Analysis of the methylation status of the KCNQ1OT and H19 genes in leukocyte DNA for the diagnosis and prognosis of Beckwith-Wiedemann syndrome. *Eur J Hum Genet* 2001; 9 (6): 409-18.

Gicquel C, Bertagna X, Schneid H, et al. Rearrangements at the 11p15 locus and overexpression of insulin-like growth factor-II gene in sporadic adrenocortical tumors. *J Clin Endocrinol Metab* 1994a; 78 (6): 1444-53.

Gicquel C, Leblond-Francillard M, Bertagna X, et al. Clonal analysis of human adrenocortical carcinomas and secreting adenomas. *Clin Endocrinol* (Oxf) 1994b; 40 (4): 465-77.

Gicquel C, Raffin-Sanson ML, Gaston V, et al. Structural and functional abnormalities at 11p15 are associated with the malignant phenotype in sporadic adrenocortical tumors: study on a series of 82 tumors. *J Clin Endocrinol Metab* 1997; 82 (8): 2559-65.

Gicquel C, Bertherat J, Le Bouc Y, Bertagna X. Pathogenesis of adrenocortical incidentalomas and genetic syndromes associated with adrenocortical neoplasms. *Endocrinol Metab Clin North Am* 2000; 29 (1): 1-13, vii.

Gicquel C, Bertagna X, Gaston V, et al. Molecular markers and long-term recurrences in a large cohort of patients with sporadic adrenocortical tumors. *Cancer Res* 2001; 61 (18): 6762-7.

Giordano TJ, Thomas DG, Kuick R, et al. Distinct transcriptional profiles of adrenocortical tumors uncovered by DNA microarray analysis. *Am J Pathol* 2003; 162 (2): 521-31.

Heppner C, Reincke M, Agarwal SK, et al. MEN1 gene analysis in sporadic adrenocortical neoplasms. *J Clin Endocrinol Metab* 1999; 84 (1): 216-9.

Hisada M, Garber JE, Fung CY, Fraumeni JF Jr., Li FP. Multiple primary cancers in families with Li-Fraumeni syndrome. *J Natl Cancer Inst* 1998; 90 (8): 606-11.

Kikuchi A. Tumor formation by genetic mutations in the components of the Wnt signalling pathway. *Cancer Sci* 2003; 94 (3): 225-9.

Kjellman M, Kallioniemi OP, Karhu R, *et al*. Genetic aberrations in adrenocortical tumors detected using comparative genomic hybridization correlate with tumor size and malignancy. *Cancer Res* 1996; 56 (18): 4219-23.

Kjellman M, Roshani L, Teh BT, *et al*. Genotyping of adrenocortical tumors: very frequent deletions of the MEN1 locus in 11q13 and of a 1-centimorgan region in 2p16. *J Clin Endocrinol Metab* 1999; 84 (2): 730-5.

Latronico AC, Pinto EM, Domenice S, *et al*. An inherited mutation outside the highly conserved DNA-binding domain of the p53 tumor suppressor protein in children and adults with sporadic adrenocortical tumors. *J Clin Endocrinol Metab* 2001; 86 (10): 4970-3.

Libe R, Bertherat J. Molecular genetics of adrenocortical tumors, from familial to sporadic diseases. *Eur J Endocrinol* 2005; 153 (4): 477-87.

Liu J, Kahri AI, Heikkila P, Voutilainen R. Ribonucleic acid expression of the clustered imprinted genes, p57KIP2, insulin-like growth factor II, and H19, in adrenal tumors and cultured adrenal cells. *J Clin Endocrinol Metab* 1997; 82 (6): 1766-71.

Logie A, Boulle N, Gaston V, *et al*. Autocrine role of IGF-II in proliferation of human adrenocortical carcinoma NCI H295R cell line. *J Mol Endocrinol* 1999; 23 (1): 23-32.

Naylor EW, Gardner EJ. Adrenal adenomas in a patient with Gardner's syndrome. *Clin Genet* 1981; 20 (1): 67-73.

Ohgaki H, Kleihues P, Heitz PU. p53 mutations in sporadic adrenocortical tumors. *Int J Cancer* 1993; 54 (3): 408-10.

Reincke M, Karl M, Travis WH, *et al*. p53 mutations in human adrenocortical neoplasms: immunohistochemical and molecular studies. *J Clin Endocrinol Metab* 1994; 78 (3): 790-94.

Ribeiro RC, Sandrini F, Figueiredo B, *et al*. An inherited p53 mutation that contributes in a tissue-specific manner to pediatric adrenal cortical carcinoma. *Proc Natl Acad Sci USA* 2001; 98 (16): 9330-5.

Schulte KM, Mengel M, Heinze M, *et al*. Complete sequencing and messenger ribonucleic acid expression analysis of the MEN I gene in adrenal cancer. *J Clin Endocrinol Metab* 2000; 85 (1): 441-8.

Sidhu S, Marsh DJ, Theodosopoulos G, *et al*. Comparative genomic hybridization analysis of adrenocortical tumors. *J Clin Endocrinol Metab* 2002; 87 (7): 3467-74.

Tissier F, Cavard C, Groussin L, *et al*. Mutations of beta-catenin in adrenocortical tumors: activation of the Wnt signaling pathway is a frequent event in both benign and malignant adrenocortical tumors. *Cancer Res* 2005; 65 (17): 7622-7.

Varley JM, McGown G, Thorncroft M, *et al*. Are there low-penetrance TP53 Alleles? evidence from childhood adrenocortical tumors. *Am J Hum Genet* 1999; 65 (4): 995-1006.

Weber MM, Auernhammer CJ, Kiess W, Engelhardt D. Insulin-like growth factor receptors in normal and tumorous adult human adrenocortical glands. *Eur J Endocrinol* 1997; 136 (3): 296-303.

Zhao J, Speel EJ, Muletta-Feurer S, *et al*. Analysis of genomic alterations in sporadic adrenocortical lesions. Gain of chromosome 17 is an early event in adrenocortical tumorigenesis. *Am J Pathol* 1999; 155 (4): 1039-45.

Pathological pattern of adrenal cortical carcinoma

Frédérique Tissier
Pathological Anatomy, Cochin Hospital, APHP, Paris;
Faculty of Medicine René Descartes, Univ. Paris 5, Paris;
Endocrinology Department, INSERM U567, Institut Cochin, Paris

Adrenal cortical carcinoma (ACC) is a malignant epithelial tumor of adrenal cortical cells (DeLellis, 2004). The role of the pathologist is first to diagnose adrenocortical tumor, second to differentiate malignant from benign tumor, and third to try to determine prognosis in case of malignancy. For these reasons, special recommendations have been developed for the surgical pathology report for tumors of the adrenal cortex (Lack, 1999).

Macroscopic examination and macroscopic findings

Macroscopic examination (Lack, 1999)

The following stages must be respected:

- Clinical data are necessary before dissecting the surgical specimen.

- Before weighing the tumor, adipose tissue surrounding the gland is removed to avoid overestimating the weight of the tumor, this parameter being essential for distinguishing benign from malignant tumors.

- The tumor, and the remnant adrenal are measured according to length, width and thickness (the thickness of normal cortex is around one millimeter).

- A thorough description of the tumor is carried out (lobulation, color, fibrosis, cystic degeneration, hemorrhage, necrosis), as well as of adjacent adrenal remnant (atrophic, nonvisible).

- Gross photography is taken.

- The following samples are carefully collected from fresh tumor specimen rapidly obtained after surgical resection (less than 10 minutes). Samples (2-10) are rapidly frozen in liquid nitrogen, from the tumor, adrenal remnant and adipose tissue surrounding the gland. After formalin fixing, samples of the tumor are performed: samples with both the tumor and the rim of adipose tissue surrounding it, samples at the junction of the tumor and of the adrenal remnant if the normal gland can be observed. The number of samples is evaluated by the pathologist according to the size and of the pattern of the lesion. At least one sample per centimeter.

Macroscopic findings

ACCs are generally bulky tumors (Lack, 1995), most weigh more than 100 g (Saeger, 2000), and are larger than 5-6 cm in diameter (Ross, 1990). According to several series, the average size of ACCs was 12,0 cm (Icard, 2001), 12,4 cm (King, 1979) and 14,0cm (Weiss, 1984). In more recent series, the median tumor size seems smaller: 8.0 cm (range, 3.5 to 20.0 cm) (Favia, 2001), 9.2 cm (range, 1.7 to 30 cm) (Barnett, 2000) and 12.0 cm (range, 1.7 to 35.0 cm) (Vassilopoulou-Sellin, 2001).

On section surface, ACCs appear yellow-orange *(figures 1-3)* to beige-rosy *(figure 4)*. ACCs are often lobulated due to fibrous bands separating tumor nodules *(figures 1, 2, 4, 5)*. Necrotic areas are generally present and they appear white-yellow *(figures 1, 2, 4, 6)*. Areas of hemorrhage and cystic degeneration may be observed. ACCs may appear encapsulated *(figure 3)*, adherent to adjacent structures *(figures 2, 5, 6)* or infiltrating adjacent organs such as the kidney. The remaining adrenal is generally not visible.

In short, gross findings may be different for smaller tumors that are homogenous and look benign in rare cases *(figure 3)* than for bulky, lobulated and necrotic tumors that have obvious malignant features *(figures 1, 2, 4, 5, 6)* (Lack, 1995).

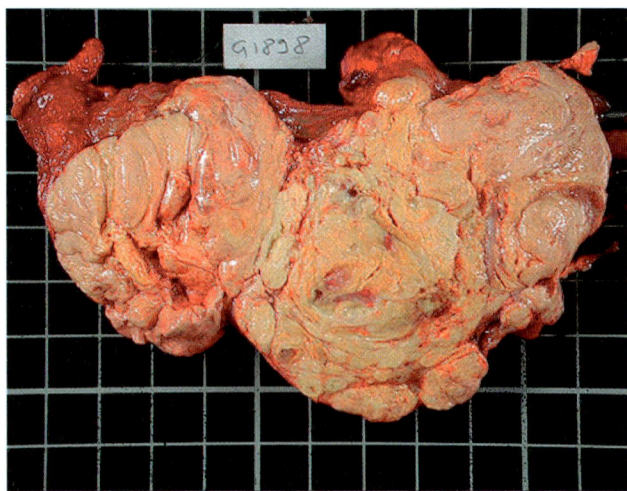

Figure 1. Macroscopic pattern: yellow-orange lobulated ACC.

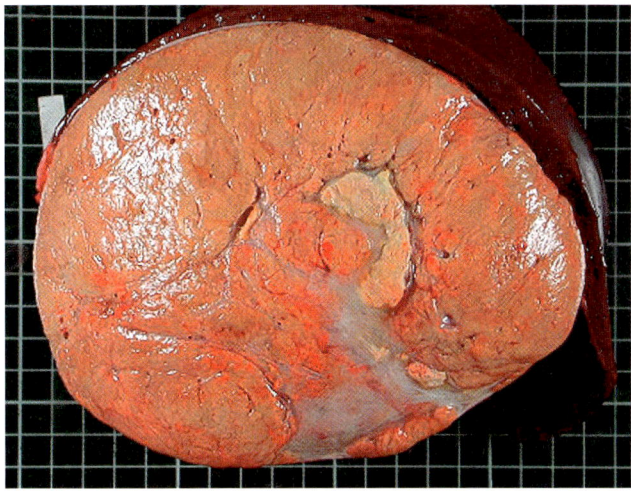

Figure 2. Macroscopic pattern: ACC adherent to the liver.

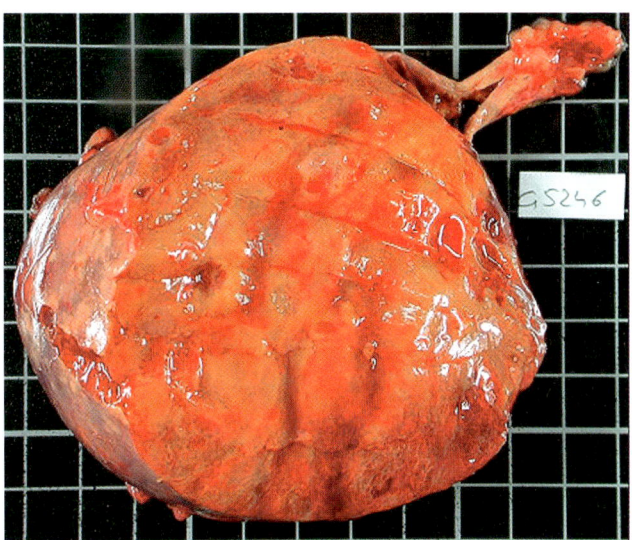

Figure 3. Macroscopic pattern: yellow-orange ACC mimicking a benign tumor.

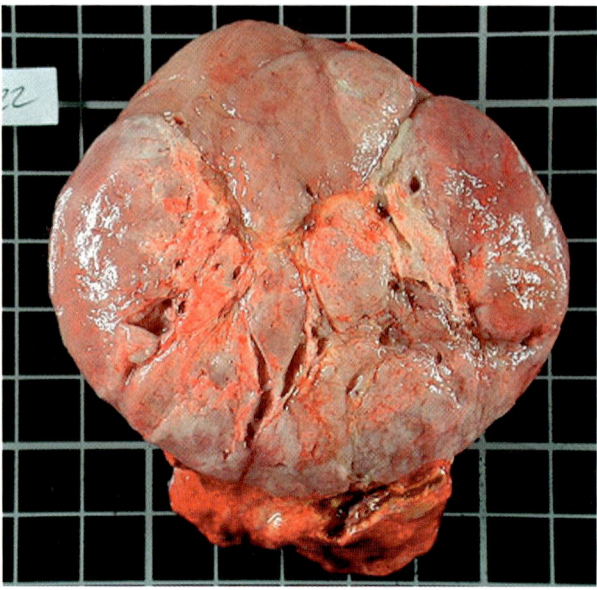

Figure 4. Macroscopic pattern: beige-rosy lobulated ACC with necrotic areas.

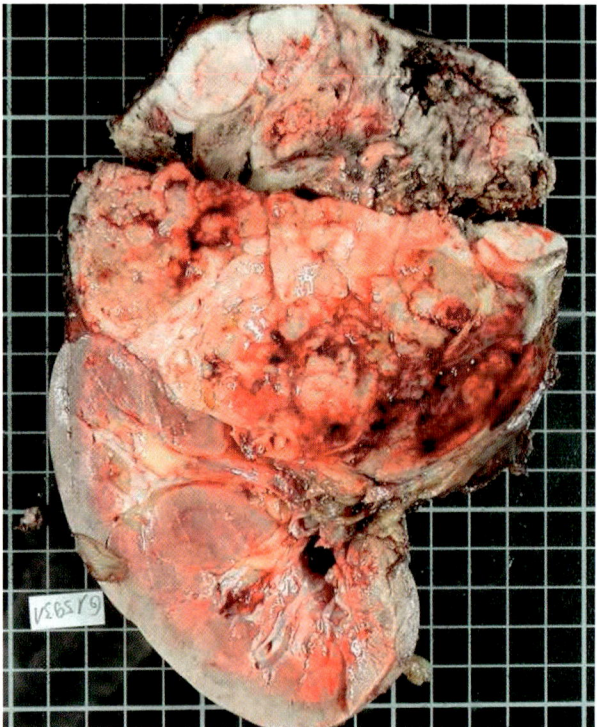

Figure 5. Macroscopic pattern: ACC adherent to the kidney and mimicking infiltration of renal parenchyma.

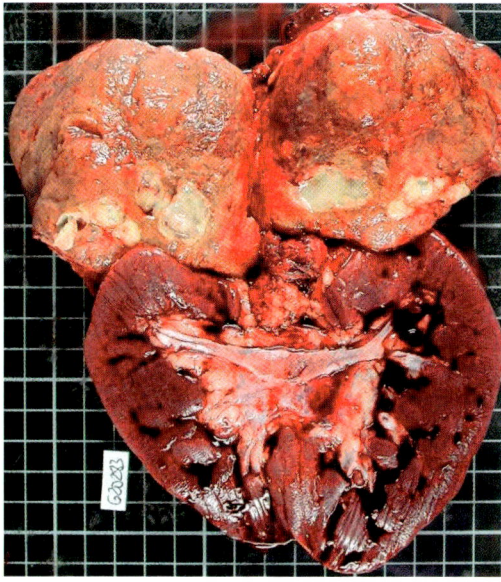

Figure 6. Macroscopic pattern: ACC adherent to the kidney.

Histological findings

Architecture

Trabecular, nesting, alveolar, diffuse or solid architectural patterns may all be observed in ACCs (Lack, 1995). The classical pattern is broad trabecular with cords of cells separated by a fine network of sinusoids *(figures 7, 8)*. Rarely, serpiginous cords or myxoid pattern are observed (Brown, 2000). Broad fibrous bands, confluent necrosis and calcification may be present *(figure 9)* (DeLellis, 2004; Lack, 1995).

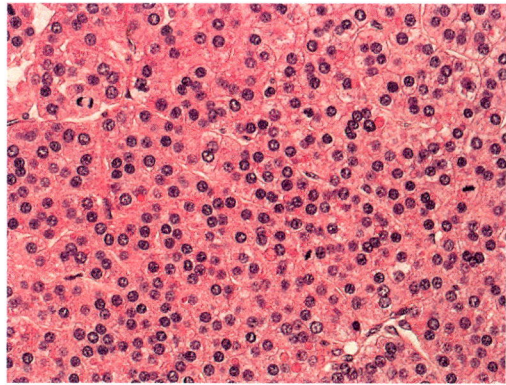

Figure 7. Histological pattern: trabeculae of eosinophilic cells (HESx200).

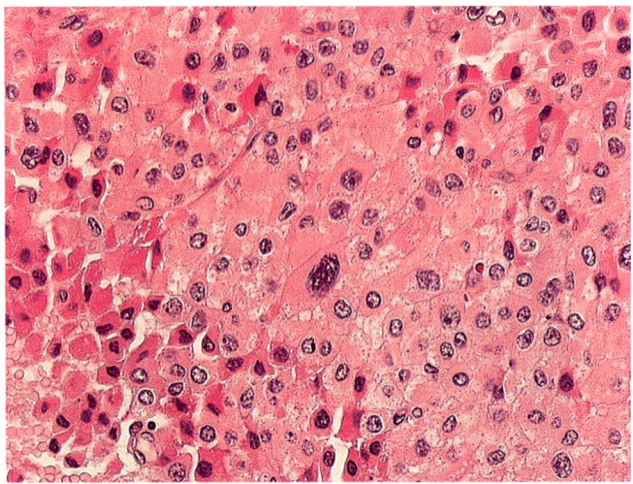

Figure 8. Histological pattern: high nuclear grade (HESx200).

Cytological pattern

Usually, ACCs present a predominance of eosinophilic compact cells depleted in lipid vacuoles *(figures 7, 8)* (DeLellis, 2004). Clear cells are rare. Nuclear pleomorphism with lobulated or multinuclear nuclei, prominent nuclear membrane and hyperchromasia, is frequent *(figures 7, 8)*. Nucleoli are conspicuous. Mitoses are generally present and mitotic rate varies widely *(figures 7, 10)* (DeLellis, 2004). Abnormal mitotic figures may be found. Variability between pathologists is frequent in the counting of mitoses and in the identification of abnormal mitotic figures (Stojadinovic, 2003).

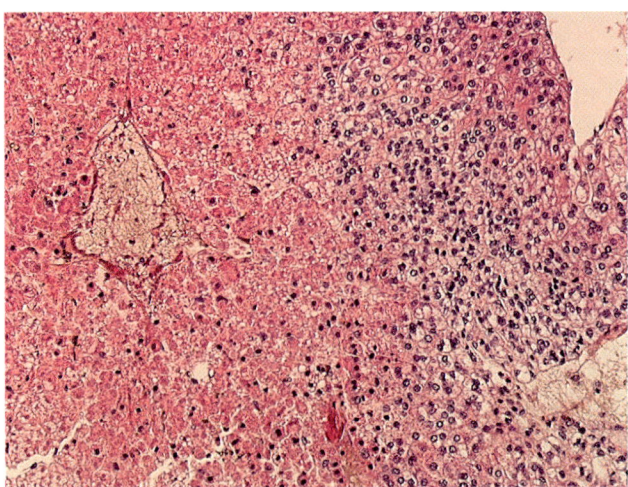

Figure 9. Histological pattern: necrosis area (HESx100).

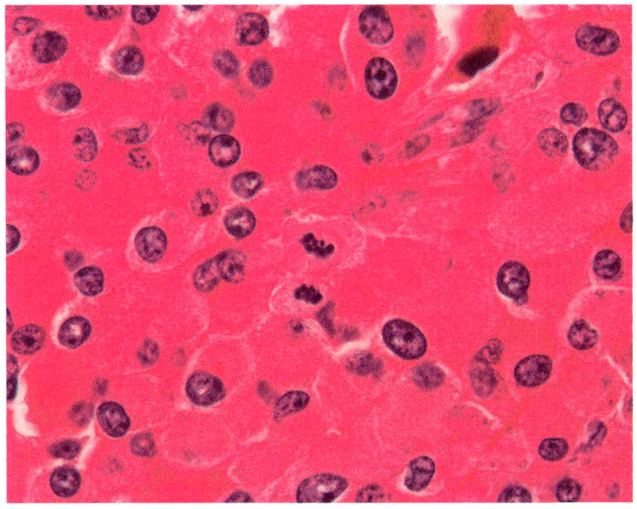

Figure 10. Histological pattern: mitoses (HESx400).

Capsular invasion and vascular invasion

Invasion of the capsule, of sinusoidal and venous vessels may be observed *(figures 11, 12, 13)*. Appraisal of capsular and vascular invasion is often difficult and may lead to discrepant results; venous or sinusoidal invasion is obvious when a vein or sinusoid internal or external to the tumor contains tumor cells within its lumen that are adherent to the vessel wall (Stojadinovic, 2003). Unequivocal capsular invasion is characterized by complete capsular penetration by tumor (Stojadinovic, 2003). Invasion of the inferior vena cava has been described (Brabrand, 1987; Ritchey, 1987). Invasion of surrounding adipose tissue or adjacent organs such as the kidney may be seen.

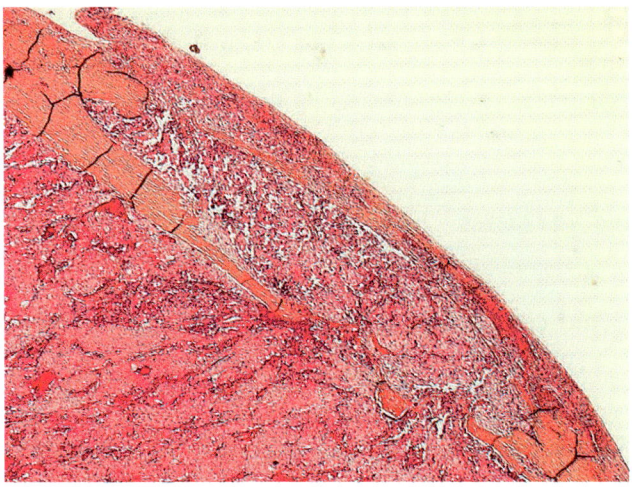

Figure 11. Histological pattern: capsular invasion (HESx25).

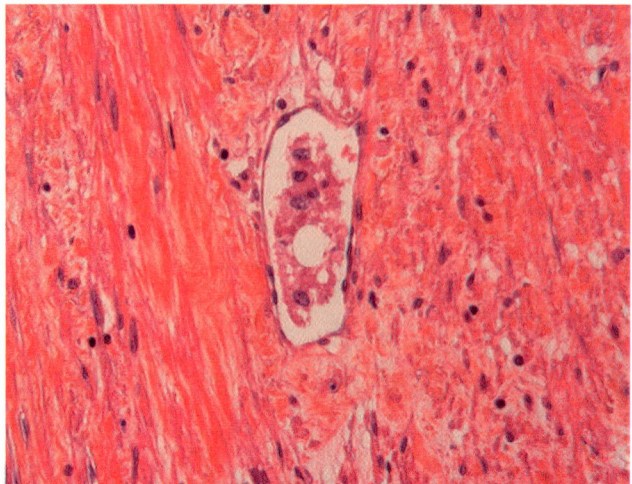

Figure 12. Histological pattern: sinusoidal invasion (HESx100).

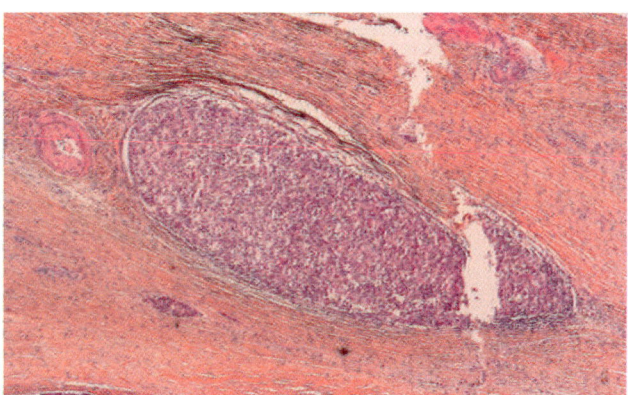

Figure 13. Histological pattern: vascular invasion (HESx25).

Rare variants

Adrenal cortical carcinoma with oncocytic features

Oncocytic ACCs have been described (el-Naggar, 1991; Hoang, 2002; Lin, 1998; Tanaka, 2004). They consist of large yellow-tan tumors. The architecture is often diffuse. Neoplastic cells present abundant eosinophilic and granular cytoplasms. Large nuclei are seen with conspicious nucleoli. Mitoses are rare (Hoang, 2002). Ultrastructurally, tumoral cells contain many mitochondria (el-Naggar, 1991). These tumors seem non-functioning (Hoang, 2002; Lin, 1998).

Adrenal cortical carcinoma with sarcomatous areas (adrenal carcinosarcoma)

Adrenal carcinosarcomas are very rare (Decorato, 1990; Fischler, 1992; Lee, 1997). They present both carcinomatous and sarcomatous elements. The sarcomatous component of the tumor may show osteogenic, chondroid or rhabdomyosarcomatous differentiation (Barksdale, 1993; Fischler, 1992).

Immunohistochemical findings

ACCs are generally negative for cytokeratin (Cote, 1990; Gaffey, 1992; Schroder, 1992) including CK 7 and CK 20 (Chu, 2000). They are generally positive for vimentin (Cote, 1990; Gaffey, 1992). ACCs are positive for Melan-A (MART-1) with a strong, diffuse cytoplasmic signal *(figure 14)* (Busam, 1998; Ghorab, 2003; Pan, 2005) and they are positive for α-inhibin, also with strong, diffuse cytoplasmic signal (Arola, 2000a; Fetsch, 1999; Pan, 2005).

Differential diagnosis

Carcinoma versus adenoma: Criteria for malignancy

For establishing the differential diagnosis between ACC and adenoma, clinical (Macfarlane, 1958), biochemical (Sidhu, 2003) and molecular criteria (Gicquel, 2001) are obviously useful, in addition to macroscopic, histological and immunohistochemical criteria.

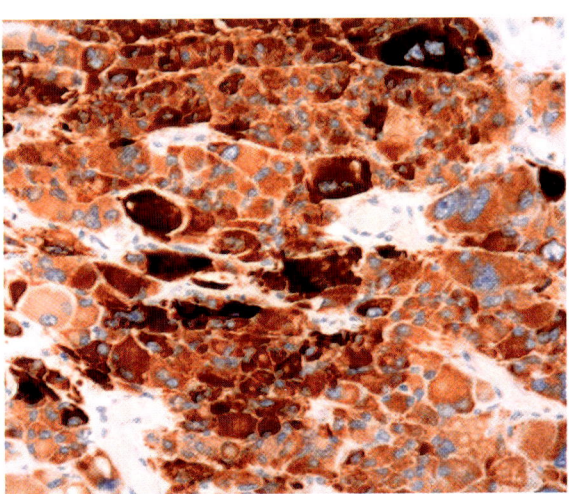

Figure 14. Immunohistochemical pattern: Melan-A (Dako, Glostrup, Denmark, HESx200).

Macroscopic criteria

Most ACCs weigh more than 100 g and are usually larger than 5-6 cm in diameter, whereas benign adrenocortical tumors weigh less than 50 g and are smaller than 5-6 cm (Lack, 1995; Ross, 1990). ACCs are often lobulated (Lack, 1995).

Histological criteria

A combination of histological features are helpful in determining malignancy of an adrenocortical tumor and several systems have been proposed to discriminate between ACC and adenoma *(tables I-IV)* (Aubert, 2002; Hough, 1979; van Slooten, 1985; Weiss, 1984).

– Some features are common to all proposed systems, like necrosis and mitoses, but assessment of this last criterion differs according to the system.

– Other criteria are common to most systems, like tumor architecture, venous invasion and capsular invasion, and nuclear pleomorphism (Hough, 1979; van Slooten, 1985; Weiss, 1984).

– Some criteria are present in half of the systems as nuclear atypia (Aubert, 2002; Weiss, 1984), < 25% clear cells (Aubert, 2002; Weiss, 1984), fibrosis (Hough, 1979; van Slooten, 1985) but the method of assessment varies according to the systems.

– Some criteria are found in only one system, like extensive regressive changes such as hemorrhage and calcification (but not necrosis) (van Slooten, 1985), nuclear hyperchromasia (van Slooten, 1985) (that can be included in pleomorphism in the Hough system (Hough, 1979)), abnormal nucleoli (van Slooten, 1985) (that can be included in nuclear atypia in the Weiss system (Weiss, 1984) or the Aubert system (Aubert, 2002)).

– In addition, nonhistologic criteria such as clinical, biochemical and macroscopic features are included in the Hough system (Hough, 1979).

Immunohistochemical criteria

The Ki-67 proliferation index may be useful as a diagnostic marker for malignancy in adrenocortical tumors (Arola, 2000b; Bernini, 2002; Kiiveri, 2005; McNicol, 1997b; Nakazumi, 1998; Stojadinovic, 2003; Terzolo, 2001; Wachenfeld, 2001). The labelling rates that distinguish malignant from benign tumors show wide variations between authors: from 12 to 63% in malignant and from 0.5 to 2.0% in benign tumors (Bernini, 2002; Nakazumi, 1998; Terzolo, 2001; Wachenfeld, 2001). Occasional ACCs may have a low proliferation index, such as a benign tumor (Stojadinovic, 2003). The Ki-67 labelling index has been shown to be higher in hormonally inactive ACCs (Arola, 2000b).

P53 immunohistochemistry may be of some help to diagnose ACCs (McNicol, 1997a; McNicol, 1997b; Wachenfeld, 2001). Although it has good specificity for ACCs, some studies find only a low prevalence of ACCs overexpressing p53 (Barzon, 2001; Stojadinovic, 2003). It should be noted that the criteria for p53 overexpression varies between 1% (Wachenfeld, 2001) to 5% of tumor cells (Stojadinovic, 2002).

Table I. Histopathological criteria proposed by Weiss (Weiss, 1984) for establishing differential diagnosis between ACC and adenoma. A score of three or more correlates with malignancy.

Histological criteria	Weighted Value (0 or 1)	
High nuclear grade	1 and 2 0	3 and 4 1
Mitoses	≤ 5 per 50 HPF 0	≥ 6 per 50 HPF 1
Abnormal mitosis	Absent 0	Present 1
Clear cells	> 25% 0	≤ 25% 1
Diffuse architecture	≤ 33% surface 0	> 33% surface 1
Necrosis	Absent 0	Present 1
Venous invasion (smooth muscle in wall)	Absent 0	Present 1
Sinusoidal invasion (no smooth muscle in wall)	Absent 0	Present 1
Capsular invasion	Absent 0	Present 1

HPF: High Power Fields

Table II. Histopathological criteria proposed by Van Slooten *et al.* (van Slooten, 1985) for establishing differential diagnosis between ACC and adenoma. Histological index > 8 correlates with malignancy.

Histological criteria	Weighted Value (0 to 9)	
Extensive regressive changes (necrosis, hemorrhage, fibrosis, calcification)	Absent 0	Present 5,7
Loss of normal structure	Absent 0	Present 1,6
Nuclear atypia	Absent or slight 0	Moderate/strong 2,1
Nuclear hyperchromasia atypia	Absent or slight 0	Moderate/marked 2,6
Abnormal nucleoli	Absent 0	Present 4,1
Mitotic activity	≤ 2 per 10 HPF 0	> 2 per 10 HPF 9,0
Vascular and/or capsular invasion	Absent 0	Present 3,3

HPF: High Power Fields

Table III. Histopathological criteria proposed by Hough *et al.* (Hough, 1979) for establishing differential diagnosis between ACC and adenoma. The mean histological index of malignant tumors is 2,91, of indeterminate tumors 1,00 and of benign tumors 0,17.

Criteria	Weighted Value (0 to 2)	
NONHISTOLOGICAL CRITERIA		
Tumor mass	< 100g 0	> 100g 0,60
Urinary 17-ketosteroids (mg/g creatinine per 24 hours)	< 10 0	> 10 0,30
Response to ACTH administration (17-hydroxysteroids increased twofold after 50μg ACTH intravenous)	Negative 0	Positive 0,42
Cushing syndrome with virilism, virilism alone, or no clinical syndrome	Absent 0	Present 0,42
Weight loss in last three months in pounds	< 10 0	> 10 2,00
HISTOLOGICAL CRITERIA		
Diffuse growth pattern (sheets without organization into trabeculae or alveolae)	Absent 0	Present 0,92
Vascular invasion	Absent 0	Present 0,92
Tumor cell Necrosis	Absent or focal 0	Wide-spread 0,69
Broad fibrous bands	Absent 0	Present 1,00
Capsular invasion	Absent 0	Present 0,37
Mitotic index (number of mitoses in 100 HPF divided by 10)	< 1 0	> 1 0,60
Pleomorphism (nuclei with high N/C ratio, marked variation in nuclear characteristics, giant cells with hyperchromatic nuclei)	Absent or slight 0	Marked 0,39

HPF: High Power Fields, N/C: nuclear/cytoplasmic

IGF-2 expression, evaluated by immunohistochemistry, may also be of value and is higher in ACCs than in adenomas (Erickson, 2001).

G1 cyclins, particularly cyclin E, play an important role in carcinogenesis (Tissier, 2004). Cyclin E overexpression is diagnosed when nuclear expression is demonstrated in more than 5% of tumors cells. In adrenocortical tumors, it has been shown that cyclin E overexpression is associated with malignancy *(figure 15)* (Tissier, 2004). In this recent study, the median was 17.5% (range, 0 to 80%) in ACCs compared to 5% (range: 0 to 70%) in benign tumors.

Table IV. Modification of the Weiss system proposed by Aubert *et al.* (Aubert, 2002) for establishing differential diagnosis between ACC and adenoma. A score of three or more correlates with malignancy.

Histological criteria	Weighted Value (0 to 2)	
Mitotic rate	≤ 5 per 50 HPF 0	≥ 6 per 50 HPF 2
Abnormal mitoses	Absent 0	Present 1
Clear cells	> 25% 0	≤ 25% 2
Necrosis	Absent 0	Present 1
Capsular invasion	Absent 0	Present 1

HPF: High Power Fields

The Wnt signaling pathway, particularly β-catenin, also plays a central role in carcinogenesis (Tissier, 2005). A hallmark of active β-catenin signaling is cytoplasmic/nuclear immunostaining for β-catenin. Abnormal and diffuse nuclear β-catenin immunostaining has been demonstrated in ACCs, whereas it is normal or cytoplasmic and focal in benign tumors *(figure 16)* (Tissier, 2005).

Adrenal cortical carcinoma versus pheochromocytoma

A combination of clinical, biochemical findings and histological features can generally establish differential diagnosis between ACC and pheochromocytoma. Sometimes ACC and pheochromocytoma may have overlapping histological features and chromogranin A, α-inhibin and Melan-A are useful to differentiate these tumors. Chromogranin A is almost always positive in pheochromocytoma and is negative in ACC (Jorda, 2002). Both tumors are generally negative for cytokeratins (Jorda, 2002).

Adrenal cortical carcinoma versus metastasis

Because of their overlapping histological features, the main differential diagnoses with ACC include hepatocellular carcinoma and renal cell carcinoma metastases (Pan, 2005). Immunohistochemistry is essential to differentiate between these tumors. Thus, Hep Par (anti-hepatocyte antibody), CD10, cytokeratins, vimentin, α-inhibin and Melan-A are useful. Cytokeratins are generally positive in hepatocellular carcinomas and in renal cell carcinomas, whereas they are generally negative in ACCs (Cote, 1990; Gaffey, 1992; Pan, 2005; Schroder, 1992). Hep Par is positive in most hepatocellular carcinomas and CD10 is positive in many renal cell carcinomas. Melan-A and α-inhibin are generally negative in hepatocellular carcinomas and in renal cell carcinomas, and they are generally positive in ACCs (Arola, 2000a; Busam, 1998; Fetsch, 1999; Pan, 2005). Vimentin is generally negative in hepatocellular carcinomas but often positive in renal cell carcinomas and positive in ACCs (Cote, 1990; Gaffey, 1992).

Staging

ACCs are classified according to several features including size, local invasion, metastases. The MacFarlane classification is frequently used *(table V)* (Macfarlane, 1958).

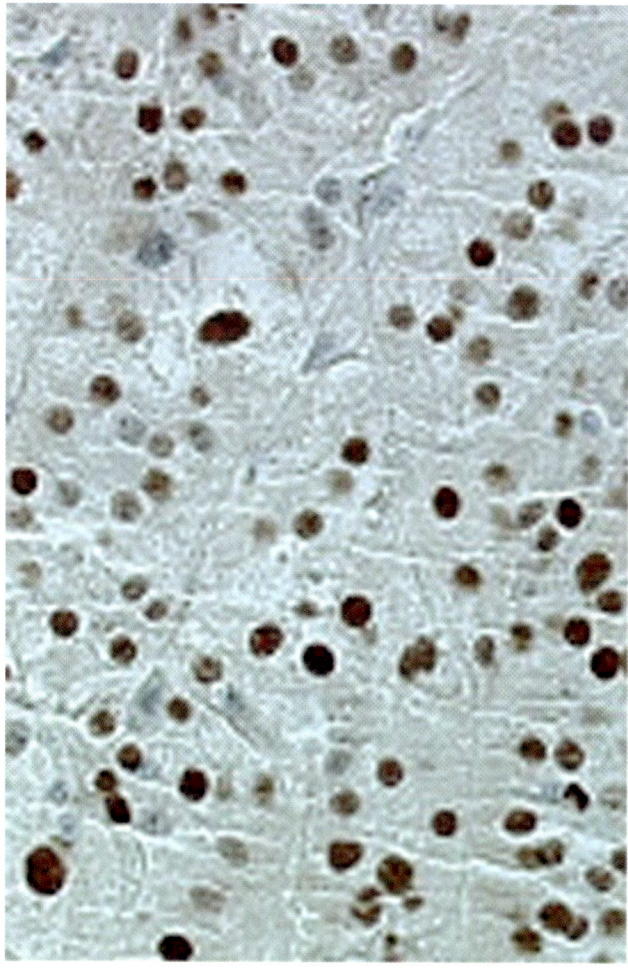

Figure 15. Immunohistochemical pattern: cyclin E (Santa Cruz, CA, USA, HESx400).

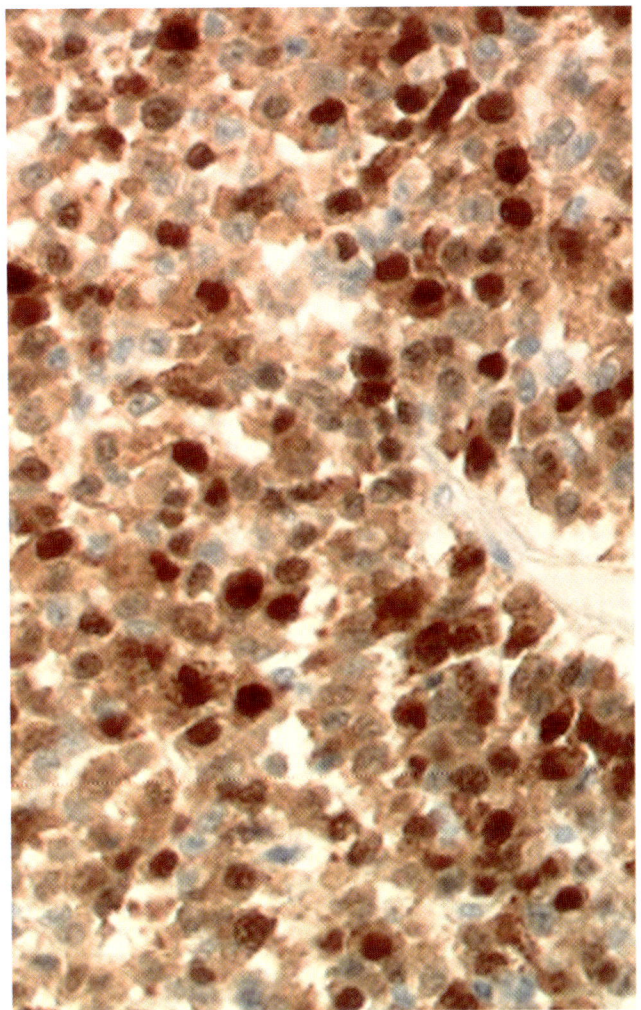

Figure 16. Immunohistochemical pattern: β-catenin (BD Biosciences, San Diego, CA, HESx400).

Table V. McFarlane Classification.

Stage I	Tumor ≤ 5 cm
Stage II	Tumor > 5 cm
Stage III	Any tumor size and mobile nodes or Infiltration locally reaching neighbouring organs and no lymph node
Stage IV	Invasion of neighbouring organs or any tumor size and fixed nodes or any tumor size, any lymph nodes and metastasis

Grading

It has been proposed that ACCs with more than 20 mitoses per 50 high power field be considered as high grade and tumors with 20 mitoses or less as low grade (Weiss, 1989).

Pathological pattern and prognosis

For assessing the prognosis of an ACCs, clinical (Macfarlane, 1958), biochemical (Sidhu, 2003), macroscopic, histological, immunohistochemical and molecular criteria (Gicquel, 2001) have to be combined.

On a pathological level, tumor size (Harrison, 1999), mitotic count (Harrison, 1999; Weiss, 1989), Ki-67 (Terzolo, 2001) and cyclin E (Tissier, 2004) have been found to correlate with shorter survival. It has been found that patients with tumor larger than 12 cm had a worse prognosis than patients with smaller tumors (Harrison, 1999). The same observation has been made for mitotic rate, but the methods of counting vary according to studies: $\geq 6/10$ high-power fields (Harrison, 1999) or $> 20/50$ high-power fields (Weiss, 1989). Some studies showed that there was no significant difference in survival between carcinomas with low Ki-67 index and those with higher index (Nakazumi, 1998) but disease-free survival was longer in the last group (McNicol, 1997b). On the other hand, other studies found a significant difference in survival (Terzolo, 2001). Abnormal p53 expression has not been shown to have any significant prognostic value in carcinoma (McNicol, 1997a). Cyclin E overexpression has been associated with poor prognostic significance in adrenocortical tumors (Tissier, 2004).

References

Arola J, Liu J, Heikkila P, Ilvesmaki V, Salmenkivi K, Voutilainen R, Kahri AI. Expression of inhibin alpha in adrenocortical tumors reflects the hormonal status of the neoplasm. *J Endocrinol* 2000; 165: 223-9.

Arola J, Salmenkivi K, Liu J, Kahri AI, Heikkila P. p53 and Ki67 in Adrenocortical tumors. *Endocr Res* 2000b; 26: 861-5.

Aubert S, Wacrenier A, Leroy X, Devos P, Carnaille B, Proye C, Wemeau JL, Lecomte-Houcke M, Leteurtre E. Weiss system revisited: a clinicopathologic and immunohistochemical study of 49 adrenocortical tumors. *Am J Surg Pathol* 2002; 26: 1612-9.

Barksdale SK, Marincola FM, Jaffe G. Carcinosarcoma of the adrenal cortex presenting with mineralocorticoid excess. *Am J Surg Pathol* 1993; 17: 941-5.

Barnett CC Jr., Varma DG, El-Naggar AK, Dackiw AP, Porter GA, Pearson AS, Kudelka AP, Gagel RF, Evans DB, Lee JE. Limitations of size as a criterion in the evaluation of adrenal tumors. *Surgery* 2000; 128: 973-982; discussion 982-973.

Barzon L, Chilosi M, Fallo F, Martignoni G, Montagna L, Palu G, Boscaro M. Molecular analysis of CDKN1C and TP53 in sporadic adrenal tumors. *Eur J Endocrinol* 2001; 145: 207-12.

Bernini GP, Moretti A, Viacava P, Bonadio AG, Iacconi P, Miccoli P, Salvetti A. Apoptosis control and proliferation marker in human normal and neoplastic adrenocortical tissues. *Br J Cancer* 2002; 86: 1561-5.

Brabrand K, Soreide JA. Adrenal cortical carcinoma with invasion into the inferior vena cava. *Br J Surg* 1987; 74: 598-9.

Brown FM, Gaffey TA, Wold LE, Lloyd RV. Myxoid neoplasms of the adrenal cortex: a rare histologic variant. *Am J Surg Pathol* 2000; 24: 396-401.

Busam KJ, Iversen K, Coplan KA, Old LJ, Stockert E, Chen YT, McGregor D, Jungbluth A. Immunoreactivity for A103, an antibody to melan-A (Mart-1), in adrenocortical and other steroid tumors. *Am J Surg Pathol* 1998; 22: 57-63.

Chu P, Wu E, Weiss LM. Cytokeratin 7 and cytokeratin 20 expression in epithelial neoplasms: a survey of 435 cases. *Mod Pathol* 2000; 13: 962-72.

Cote RJ, Cordon-Cardo C, Reuter VE, Rosen PP. Immunopathology of adrenal and renal cortical tumors. Coordinated change in antigen expression is associated with neoplastic conversion in the adrenal cortex. *Am J Pathol* 1990; 136: 1077-84.

Decorato JW, Gruber H, Petti M, Levowitz BS. Adrenal carcinosarcoma. *J Surg Oncol* 1990; 45: 134-6.

DeLellis RA, Lloyd RV, Heitz PU, Eng C. Pathology and Genetics. Tumors of Endocrine Organs. World Health Organization Classification of Tumors. 2004.

el-Naggar AK, Evans DB, Mackay B. Oncocytic adrenal cortical carcinoma. *Ultrastruct Pathol* 1991; 15: 549-56.

Erickson LA, Jin L, Sebo TJ, Lohse C, Pankratz VS, Kendrick ML, van Heerden JA, Thompson GB, Grant CS, Lloyd RV. Pathologic features and expression of insulin-like growth factor-2 in adrenocortical neoplasms. *Endocr Pathol* 2001; 12: 429-35.

Favia G, Lumachi F, D'Amico DF. Adrenocortical carcinoma: is prognosis different in nonfunctioning tumors? results of surgical treatment in 31 patients. *World J Surg* 2001; 25: 735-8.

Fetsch PA, Powers CN, Zakowski MF, Abati A. Anti-alpha-inhibin: marker of choice for the consistent distinction between adrenocortical carcinoma and renal cell carcinoma in fine-needle aspiration. *Cancer* 1999; 87: 168-72.

Fischler DF, Nunez C, Levin HS, McMahon JT, Sheeler LR, Adelstein DJ. Adrenal carcinosarcoma presenting in a woman with clinical signs of virilization. A case report with immunohistochemical and ultrastructural findings. *Am J Surg Pathol* 1992; 16: 626-31.

Gaffey MJ, Traweek ST, Mills SE, Travis WD, Lack EE, Medeiros LJ, Weiss LM. Cytokeratin expression in adrenocortical neoplasia: an immunohistochemical and biochemical study with implications for the differential diagnosis of adrenocortical, hepatocellular, and renal cell carcinoma. *Hum Pathol* 1992; 23: 144-53.

Ghorab Z, Jorda M, Ganjei P, Nadji M. Melan A (A103) is expressed in adrenocortical neoplasms but not in renal cell and hepatocellular carcinomas. *Appl Immunohistochem Mol Morphol* 2003; 11: 330-3.

Gicquel C, Bertagna X, Gaston V, Coste J, Louvel A, Baudin E, Bertherat J, Chapuis Y, Duclos JM, Schlumberger M, et al. Molecular markers and long-term recurrences in a large cohort of patients with sporadic adrenocortical tumors. *Cancer Res* 2001; 61: 6762-7.

Harrison LE, Gaudin PB, Brennan MF. Pathologic features of prognostic significance for adrenocortical carcinoma after curative resection. *Arch Surg* 1999; 134: 181-5.

Hoang MP, Ayala AG, Albores-Saavedra J. Oncocytic adrenocortical carcinoma: a morphologic, immunohistochemical and ultrastructural study of four cases. *Mod Pathol* 2002; 15: 973-8.

Hough AJ, Hollifield JW, Page DL, Hartmann WH. Prognostic factors in adrenal cortical tumors. A mathematical analysis of clinical and morphologic data. *Am J Clin Pathol* 1979; 72: 390-9.

Icard P, Goudet P, Charpenay C, Andreassian B, Carnaille B, Chapuis Y, Cougard P, Henry JF, Proye C. Adrenocortical carcinomas: surgical trends and results of a 253-patient series from the French Association of Endocrine Surgeons study group. *World J Surg* 2001; 25: 891-7.

Jorda M, De MB, Nadji M. Calretinin and inhibin are useful in separating adrenocortical neoplasms from pheochromocytomas. *Appl Immunohistochem Mol Morphol* 2002; 10: 67-70.

Kiiveri S, Liu J, Arola J, Heikkila P, Kuulasmaa T, Lehtonen E, Voutilainen R, Heikinheimo M. Transcription factors GATA-6, SF-1, and cell proliferation in human adrenocortical tumors. *Mol Cell Endocrinol* 2005; 233: 47-56.

King DR, Lack EE. Adrenal cortical carcinoma: a clinical and pathologic study of 49 cases. *Cancer* 1979; 44: 239-44.

Lack EE. Tumors of the adrenal gland and extra-adrenal paraganglia. Atlas of tumor pathology, Washington, DC. 1995.

Lack EE. Recommendations for the reporting of tumors of the adrenal cortex and medulla. Association of Directors of Anatomic and Surgical Pathology. *Virchows Arch* 1999; 435: 87-91.

Lee MS, Park IA, Chi JG, Ham EK, Lee KC, Lee CW. Adrenal carcinosarcoma - a case report. *J Korean Med Sci* 1997; 12: 374-7.

Lin BT, Bonsib SM, Mierau GW, Weiss LM, Medeiros LJ. Oncocytic adrenocortical neoplasms: a report of seven cases and review of the literature. *Am J Surg Pathol* 1998; 22: 603-14.

Macfarlane DA. Cancer of the adrenal cortex; the natural history, prognosis and treatment in a study of fifty-five cases. *Ann R Coll Surg Engl* 1958; 23: 155-86.

McNicol AM, Nolan CE, Struthers AJ, Farquharson MA, Hermans J, Haak HR. Expression of p53 in adrenocortical tumors: clinicopathological correlations. *J Pathol* 1997a; 181: 146-52.

McNicol AM, Struthers AL, Nolan CE, Hermans J, Haak HR. Proliferation in Adrenocortical Tumors: Correlation with Clinical Outcome and p53 Status. *Endocr Pathol* 1997b; 8: 29-36.

Nakazumi H, Sasano H, Iino K, Ohashi Y, Orikasa S. Expression of cell cycle inhibitor p27 and Ki-67 in human adrenocortical neoplasms. *Mod Pathol* 1998; 11: 1165-70.

Pan CC, Chen PC, Tsay SH, Ho DM. Differential immunoprofiles of hepatocellular carcinoma, renal cell carcinoma, and adrenocortical carcinoma: a systemic immunohistochemical survey using tissue array technique. *Appl Immunohistochem Mol Morphol* 2005; 13: 347-52.

Ritchey ML, Kinard R, Novicki DE. Adrenal tumors: involvement of the inferior vena cava. *J Urol* 1987; 138: 1134-6.

Ross NS, Aron DC. Hormonal evaluation of the patient with an incidentally discovered adrenal mass. *N Engl J Med* 1990; 323: 1401-5.

Saeger W. Histopathological classification of adrenal tumors. *Eur J Clin Invest* 2000; 30 (Suppl 3): 58-62.

Schroder S, Padberg BC, Achilles E, Holl K, Dralle H, Kloppel G. Immunocytochemistry in adrenocortical tumors: a clinicomorphological study of 72 neoplasms. *Virchows Arch A Pathol Anat Histopathol* 1992; 420: 65-70.

Sidhu S, Gicquel C, Bambach CP, Campbell P, Magarey C, Robinson BG, Delbridge LW. Clinical and molecular aspects of adrenocortical tumourigenesis. *ANZ J Surg* 2003; 73: 727-38.

Stojadinovic A, Brennan MF, Hoos A, Omeroglu A, Leung DH, Dudas ME, Nissan A, Cordon-Cardo C, Ghossein RA. Adrenocortical adenoma and carcinoma: histopathological and molecular comparative analysis. *Mod Pathol* 2003; 16: 742-51.

Stojadinovic A, Ghossein RA, Hoos A, Nissan A, Marshall D, Dudas M, Cordon-Cardo C, Jaques DP, Brennan MF. Adrenocortical carcinoma: clinical, morphologic, and molecular characterization. *J Clin Oncol* 2002; 20: 941-50.

Tanaka K, Kumano Y, Kanomata N, Takeda M, Hara I, Fujisawa M, Kawabata G, Kamidono S. Oncocytic adrenocortical carcinoma. *Urology* 2004; 64: 376-7.

Terzolo M, Boccuzzi A, Bovio S, Cappia S, De Giuli P, Ali A, Paccotti P, Porpiglia F, Fontana D, Angeli A. Immunohistochemical assessment of Ki-67 in the differential diagnosis of adrenocortical tumors. *Urology* 2001; 57: 176-82.

Tissier F, Cavard C, Groussin L, Perlemoine K, Fumey G, Hagnere AM, Rene-Corail F, Jullian E, Gicquel C, Bertagna X, *et al*. Mutations of beta-catenin in adrenocortical tumors: activation of the Wnt signaling pathway is a frequent event in both benign and malignant adrenocortical tumors. *Cancer Res* 2005; 65: 7622-7.

Tissier F, Louvel A, Grabar S, Hagnere AM, Bertherat J, Vacher-Lavenu MC, Dousset B, Chapuis Y, Bertagna X, Gicquel C. Cyclin E correlates with malignancy and adverse prognosis in adrenocortical tumors. *Eur J Endocrinol* 2004; 150: 809-17.

van Slooten H, Schaberg A, Smeenk D, Moolenaar AJ. Morphologic characteristics of benign and malignant adrenocortical tumors. *Cancer* 1985; 55: 766-73.

Vassilopoulou-Sellin R, Schultz PN. Adrenocortical carcinoma. Clinical outcome at the end of the 20th century. *Cancer* 2001; 92: 1113-21.

Wachenfeld C, Beuschlein F, Zwermann O, Mora P, Fassnacht M, Allolio B, Reincke M. Discerning malignancy in adrenocortical tumors: are molecular markers useful? *Eur J Endocrinol* 2001; 145: 335-41.

Weiss LM. Comparative histologic study of 43 metastasizing and nonmetastasizing adrenocortical tumors. *Am J Surg Pathol* 1984; 8: 163-9.

Weiss LM, Medeiros LJ, Vickery AL Jr. Pathologic features of prognostic significance in adrenocortical carcinoma. *Am J Surg Pathol* 1989; 13: 202-6.

Imaging in adrenal cortical carcinoma

Paul Legmann, Stéphane Silvera
Radiology Department, Cochin Hospital, Faculty of Medicine René Descartes, Univ. Paris 5

The development of cross sectional imaging has advanced considerably the course of investigation of patients with a suspected adrenal pathology. Previous more invasive techniques such as arteriography, veinography and biopsy are now rarely used due to improvement of accuracy in CT and MRI in evaluating adrenal gland (Krestin, 1991; Schwartz, 1996).

The adrenal gland is a common site of disease and detection of adrenal masses has become more frequent. The adrenal glands are also imaged to localize disorders indicated by abnormal biochemistry. In both cases, imaging plays a critical role not only in the detection of adrenal abnormalities but also in characterizing them as benign or malignant (Outwater, 1995; Szolar, 1997). Imaging also contributes to the detection of local invasion and/or of distant metastases, and thus to the definition of ACC (Adrenal Cortical Carcinoma) stages.

Anatomy

The adrenal glands have two distinct areas: an inner medulla that is derived from the neural crest makes up only 10% of the gland and is almost entirely within the body of the gland, and an outer cortex derived from the mesoderm which constitutes about 90% of the gland and is located in the body and the limbs of the glands.

The outer zone of the cortex: the *zona glomerulosa*, secretes mineralocorticoids (aldosterone) which control salt and water metabolism. The inner cortical zones: the *zona fasciculata* and *zona reticularis,* secrete glucocorticoids and androgens responding to pituitary ACTH which is in turn inhibited by cortisol.

The *medulla* contains chromaffin cells which produce catecholamines: mainly adrenaline (epinephrine) and noradrenaline (norepinephrine). The medulla is almost entirely localized within the body of the adrenal gland.

The adrenal gland is named for its location adjacent to the kidneys. The normal gland weighs 5 g and has a characteristic Y, V or T shape.

The normal adrenals extend 2-4 cm in the cranio-caudal direction and the thickness of the adrenal body and limbs does not exceed 10-12 and 5-6 mm respectively.

Etiology of adrenal masses

The adrenal gland is routinely identified at abdominal CT and MR imaging examinations.

Adrenal masses are estimated to occur in 9% of the population. With the proliferation of cross-sectional imaging, detection of an incidental adrenal mass has become common. In patients with no known primary cancer, an adrenal mass is almost always a benign adenoma but requires endocrinogical evaluation. Even in oncology patients, approximately 70% of adrenal masses are benign (Dunnick, 2002).

However, the precise characterization of adrenal masses is important for pre-therapeutic staging and prognosis (Dunnick, 1996).

In a patient with a known primary cancer, particularly lung cancer, the finding of an adrenal mass is problematic since metastasis indicates advanced disease not amenable to surgical resection.

Abnormalities of the adrenal gland include primary neoplasm, metastases, haemorrhage or enlargement from external hormonal stimulation...

Adrenal masses can be divided in two categories based on whether they are hypersecretory or not (McNicholas, 1995; Otal, 1999).

Hyperfunctioning adrenal masses include pheochromocytomas, aldosteronomas (Conn's adenoma), and cortisol or androgen-producing tumors. With the exception of Conn's adenoma (which is almost always benign), they can be either benign or malignant.

Adrenal adenomas and metastases are the most common nonfunctioning adrenal masses.

Imaging methods

There are numerous imaging modalities including CT, MRI, Ultrasonography (US) and nuclear medicine that can be used to evaluate the adrenal gland. Use of CT and MRI imaging has resulted in more frequent detection of incidental adrenal lesions (Kawashima, 1998).

CT is the primary method for both detection and characterization of adrenal masses.

New approaches to characterizing adrenal masses and cross section imaging include assessing lesion size, describing morphologic criteria, measuring attenuation or signal intensity, calculating the loss ratio of enhancement and thus determining the lipid content (Bae, 2003).

CT imaging

If an adrenal mass is suspected, CT technique must include use of 3 mm collimation with the field of view targeted to the adrenal gland. A nonenhanced examination should be performed first.

Currently, two main criteria (histologic and physiologic) discriminate between adenomatous and non adenomatous adrenal masses: intracellular lipid content and vascular enhancement patterns, correlate with these features which distinguish between adenomas and non adenomas.

Adenomas typically have abundant intracytoplasmic fat and thus a low attenuation at unenhanced CT, whereas non adenomas, like metastases or primary neoplasms or pheochromocytomas, do not, and thus do not show low attenuation.

Attenuation measurement is performed with a region of interest (ROI) large enough to include 2/3 of the adrenal mass surface. Attenuation measurement thresholds used to differentiate benign from malignant lesions are set at 10 Hounsfields Units (HU), with a sensitivity of 71% and a specificity of 98% for characterizing adrenal masses. This specificity approaches 100% when other features are considered, such as size greater than 4 cm, heterogeneous density and irregular shape, and rapid change in lesion size, all indicative of a malignant mass [Boland, 1998; Gufler, 2004; Korobkin, 1996, (a)].

Although the finding of low attenuation is sufficient to characterize an adenoma, it is estimated that up to 30% of adenomas do not contain high enough lipid to have low attenuation at CT.

In addition, the majority of CT examinations, not directly intended to characterize an adrenal mass, are performed with intravenous contrast material at first (no unenhanced density value can be measured).

Therefore, the second imaging parameter used to differentiate adenomas from malignant lesions relies on differences in enhancement (Boland, 1997; Caoili, 2000; Caoili, 2002): adenomas enhance rapidly with intravenous contrast (either iodinated contrast at CT or gadolinium chelates at MRI) and wash out the agent rapidly.

Other adrenal masses can also enhance similarly, but washout of the agent is more prolonged.

This difference in washout of contrast media is used currently to differentiate benign from malignant adrenal lesions.

Dynamic contrast-enhanced CT is performed 60-80 seconds after starting the intravenous injection, then delayed images are obtained 10 minutes (Black, 2005) after injection. A useful parameter is the percentage of washout of contrast material obtained by comparing attenuation of the adrenal lesion at delayed CT with its attenuation at early acquisition.

Percentage of washout is calculated as relative with the following formula: (initial enhanced value-delayed HU value/initial enhanced value) X 100, or absolute: (initial enhanced value – delayed HU value/initial enhanced HU value – non enhanced HU) X 100.

Loss of 50% of relative attenuation value at 10 minutes and of 60% of absolute HU value is considered specific for the diagnosis of a benign adenoma.

Washout of contrast media may be more specific than attenuation measurement at unenhanced CT, especially for lipid poor adenomas (Pena, 2000; Szolar, 1998).

It is important to stress that if an adrenal lesion cannot be determined, the patient should undergo MRI or even a guided biopsy, in the case of an oncology patient.

MR imaging

Various parameters can be used to characterize adrenal masses, including T1, T2, enhancement patterns after contrast media injection and chemical shift imaging.

Signal intensity at T1 and T2 weighted sequences is not useful because of a significant overlap between benign and malignant lesions.

Enhancement pattern as a means of differentiation has shown that adenomas enhance vigorously and exhibit early wash out (Korobkin, 1996, b; Krebs, 1998; Mayo-Smith, 1995).

As intracellular lipid and rapid enhancement washout appear to be two unique features of adenomas, chemical shift imaging, an MR technique used to detect lipid within an organ, is considered the most sensitive method for differentiating adenomas from non adenomas.

Chemical shift imaging relies on the different resonance frequency rates of protons in fat and water molecules.

Fat protons are more shielded than water protons and resonate at a slower frequency.

The effect of this physical phenomenon is utilized in chemical shift imaging.

Two breath-hold gradient echo T1-weigthed sequences are performed: one with an echo time (TE) at 2.2 ms at 1.5 T with fat and water protons being out of phase, and a second with TE at 4.4 ms with fat and water protons being in phase. On out of phase images there is cancellation of signal between lipid and water, with a signal drop-off.

Thus, on out of phase sequences the adenoma with lipid content appears darker than on in phase images.

When in and out of phase images are compared, it is necessary to use the spleen as a standard for signal intensity (Hussain, 2004; Israel, 2004; Outwater, 1996).

With chemical shift technique, the sensitivity and specificity for differentiating adenomas from metastases and malignant lesions ranges from 80% to 100%, and 94% to 100%.

Chemical shift imaging is the most sensitive technique for differentiating adenomas from non adenomas and malignant lesions (Korobkin, 1995; Schwartz, 1996).

Adrenal biopsy

New imaging methods most often make it possible to avoid unnecessary biopsy.

However, when adrenal lesions cannot be accurately characterized with CT, MR imaging or PET, and if a definitive diagnosis of an adrenal mass is necessary for accurate staging, adrenal biopsy can be performed as a safe and reliable technique.

Adrenal biopsies are procedures with a high degree of accuracy (85%) and a low complication rate (3%) (Paulsen, 1995; Silverman, 1993).

CT is the method of choice for guiding the procedure. Angling the CT gantry, or the patient on the ipsilateral side down are methods used for lessening the risk of a pneumothorax.

With some patients a transhepatic approach may be used.

Adrenal cortical carcinoma

Adrenal cortical carcinoma (ACC) is a rare neoplasm of the cortex, and account for only 0.02% of malignant tumors.

A majority of these tumors are functional, occasionally with secondary symptoms caused by the hormone, such as Cushing, virilization, feminization, or much less frequently hypermineralocorticism. Cushing's syndrome is the most frequently seen clinical presentation. Adrenal carcinomas account for 5-10% of cases of Cushing's syndrome.

Other manifestations include an abdominal mass and abdominal pain (Pommier, 1992).

Adrenal carcinomas are usually large at presentation, with size ranging from 4 or 5 to 10 cm or more. About 15% of carcinomas are less than 6 cm in diameter and may resemble adenomas.

Most adrenal masses larger than 6 cm in diameter are resected, because a substantial proportion are found to be malignant and most ACCs are larger than 6 cm when they are first detected clinically.

CT

At unenhanced CT, adreno-cortical carcinomas have mean attenuation value similar to those of metastases, and significantly higher than adenomas.

In adrenal carcinoma, enhanced CT can show large and low attenuation suprarenal mass containing areas of high attenuation that are consistent with haemorrhage.

The lesion appears heterogeneous and commonly contains central necrosis and calcifications.

Contrast enhanced CT scan can show mass with heterogeneous enhancement.

On a ten or fifteen minute delayed contrast scan, the mean attenuation and a mean percentage loss of enhancement for adenomas differs significantly from that observed for adrenal cortical carcinoma *(figure 1)*.

A sensitivity of 100% and a specificity of 100% for the diagnosis of adenoma when comparing 24 adenomas with 11 cortical carcinomas has been obtained (Korobkin, 1996).

When results of CT examination are equivocal, MR imaging is the next imaging study of choice for characterising adrenal lesions (Gomez-Rivera, 2005).

MRI

Adrenal cortical carcinomas are large and appear heterogeneous and hypo-hyper intense on T1 and T2 weighted images, due to the presence of internal haemorrhage or necrosis. Haemorrhage products, mainly methemoglobin, can result in areas of high signal intensity within the lesion on T1 weighted images. Areas of necrosis also have high signal intensity on T2 weighted images *(figure 2)*.

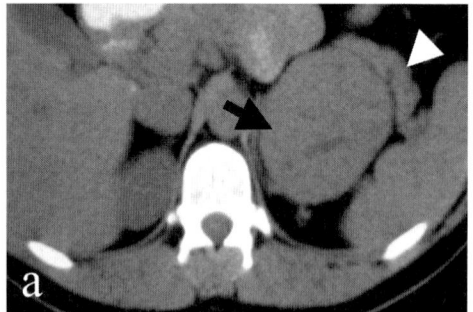
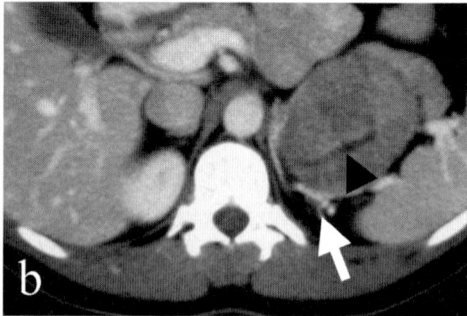
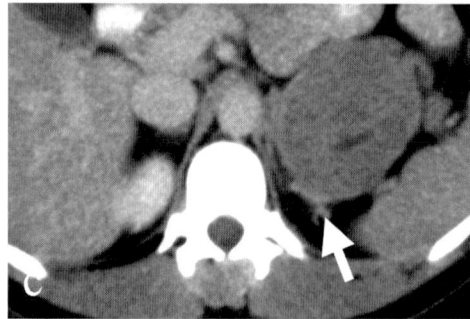

Figure 1. Adrenal cortical carcinoma in a 40-year-old-woman with Cushing syndrome. CT appearances.
(a) Axial unenhanced CT scan exhibits a large left adrenal mass (black arrow) which causes an anterior displacement of the pancreas (white arrowhead). The attenuation is measured at 41 UH, unusual for adrenal adenoma.
(b) On the 50 seconds delayed image, the mass shows low enhancement at 80 UH. Note a linear central attenuation that represents fat, confirmed at histologic analysis (black arrowhead).
(c) On the 10-minute delayed image, the attenuation is 59 UH. There is typically no wash-out between the 50 seconds delayed phase and the late delayed phase, which confirms the absence of adenoma.
Note the persistence of the left adrenal enhancement (white arrow).

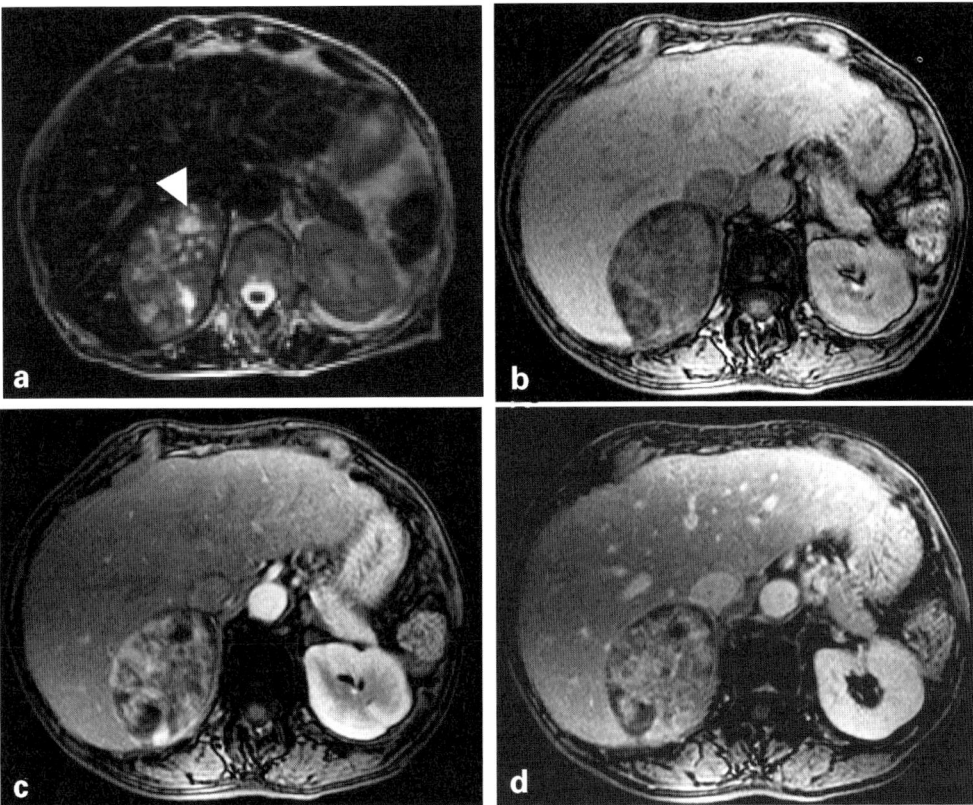

Figure 2. Cushing's syndrome due to right adrenocortical carcinoma.
MR appearances:
(a) Axial fast-spin-echo T2-weighted image shows a heterogeneous mass, with some areas on hypersignal, exhibiting areas of necrosis (white arrowhead).
(b) Axial out-of-phase image also shows a right heterogeneous mass.
(c) Dynamic enhanced image obtained 60 seconds after injection of gadolinium shows a heterogeneous enhancement of the adrenal mass.
(d) 5 minute-delayed post contrast phase shows persistence of the enhancement of the adrenal mass.

In general, metastases and carcinomas contain larger amounts of fluid than adenomas, and appear hyperintense on T2 weighted images.

Chemical shift imaging is an MR imaging technique used to detect lipid content in an organ and is the most sensitive method for differentiating adenomas from malignant lesions.

As stated above, intracellular lipid is high in most adrenal adenomas and low in malignant lesions. In adrenal masses that do not contain lipid (metastases or adrenal carcinoma) there is no significant loss of signal on out of phase images, and therefore the signal intensity of the adrenal gland is the same on in phase and out of phase images *(figure 3)*.

There is no loss of signal intensity (wash-out) on delayed post-contrast out of phase images *(figure 4)*.

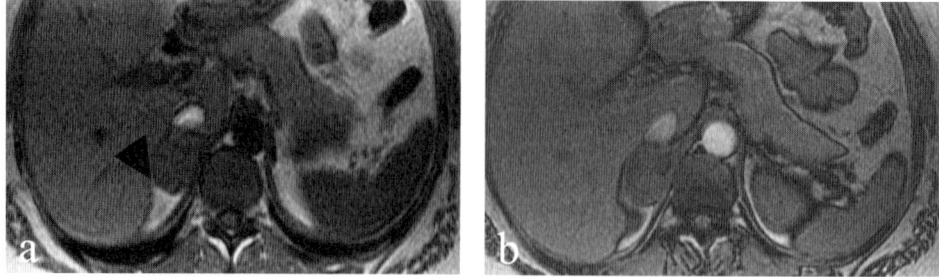

Figure 3. Right adrenocortical mass in a 39-year-old woman evaluated by MRI. Axial in-phase image shows the right adrenal mass (arrow head), homogenous with well defined margins. Note the absence of the signal dropout between the axial in-phase image (a) and the axial out-phase image (b). The signal is measured respectively at 39 UI and 34 UI.

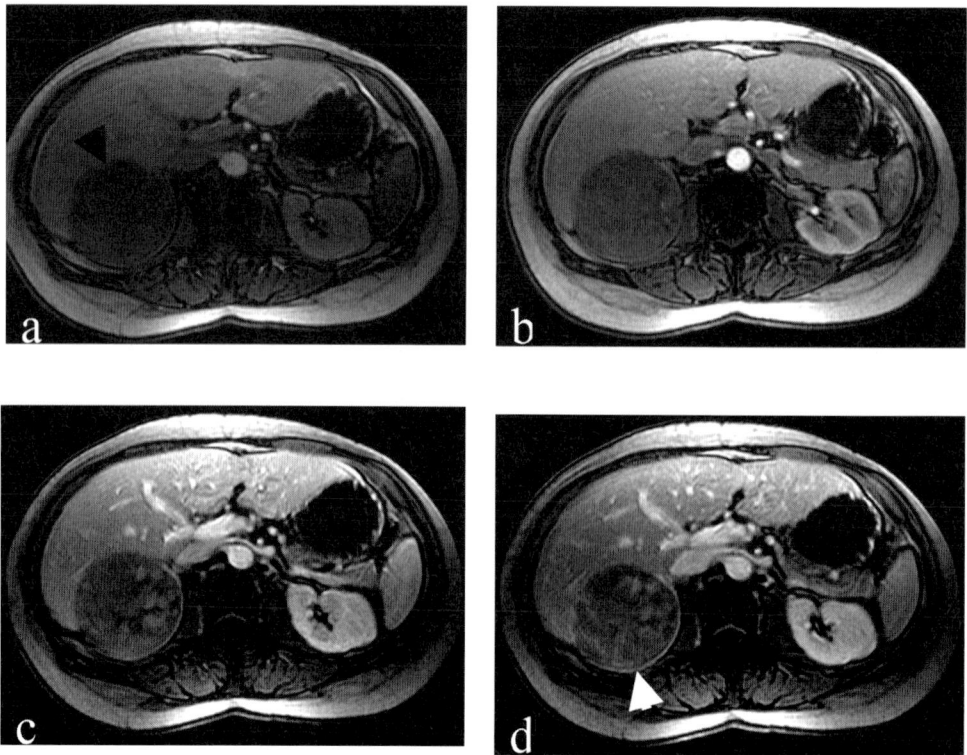

Figure 4. Right adrenocortical mass in a 53-years-old woman evaluated by MRI.
(a) Axial out-of-phase image shows a large and heterogeneous lesion (black arrow head).
Acquisition time after injection of gadolinium realized at 50 seconds (b),
3 minutes (c) and 5 minutes (d).
Dynamic out-phase images show a delay in increase of signal intensity and a peripheral capsule on the late delayed post-contrast phase (white arrowhead) (d).

But adrenal cortical carcinoma can contain areas of intracytoplasmic lipid, which result in confined loss of signal intensity on out of phase images. Large areas of necrosis are also present.

Large adrenal carcinomas tend to invade adrenal vein and inferior vena cava *(figure 5)*.

Extension of adrenal carcinoma to inferior vena cava includes potential liver metastases and lung metastases. Invasion of adjacent organs is readily demonstrated on US with Doppler studies, and MRI for which sagittal or coronal sections are obtained.

Differential diagnosis

Adrenal cortical adenomas

Adrenal adenomas causing Cushing's syndrome are usually larger than two centimetres in diameter and are visualised on CT scan.

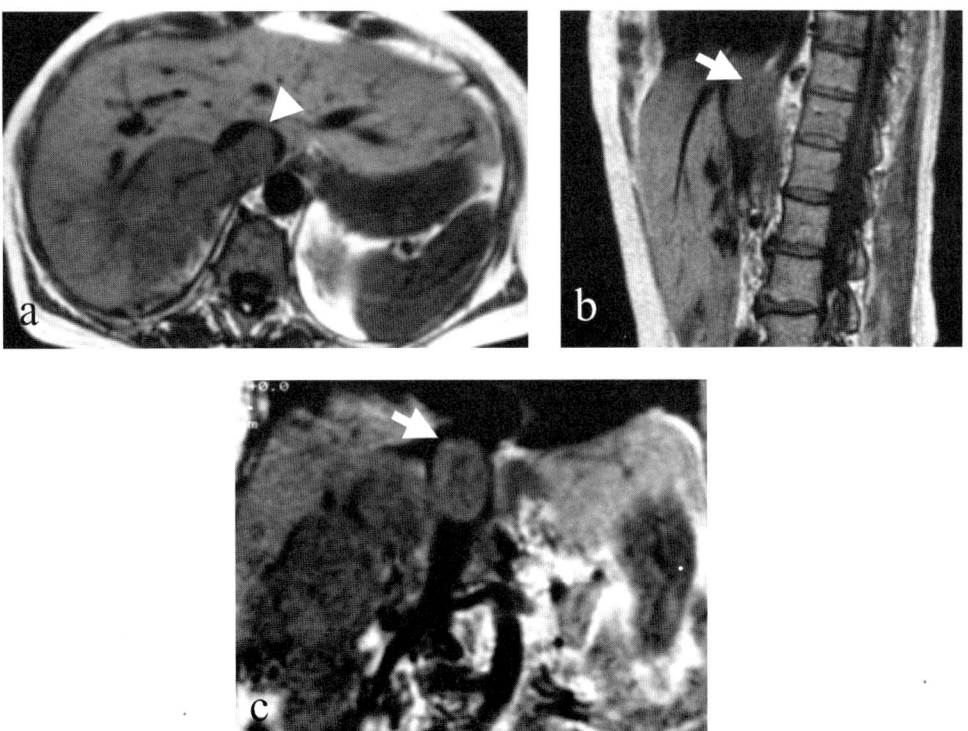

Figure 5. Right adrenocortical mass in a 50-year-old woman known for hypertension.
Axial spin-echo T1-weighted image demonstrates the right adrenal mass with extension into the inferior vena cava (IVC) (white arrowhead).
On sagittal and coronal SE T1-WI, the bud is shown in the IVC (white arrow).

In patients with adrenal mass and no evidence of endocrine hyperfunction or of an extra-adrenal primary neoplasm, differential diagnosis includes adenoma and adrenal cortical carcinoma. Rarely, collision tumor including adenoma and metastasis can occur and 18 FDG-PET/CT may be helpful (Blake, 2004).

Differentiating an adrenal mass as benign or malignant is critical in the oncologic patient.

CT imaging findings are helpful in differentiating benign from malignant lesion.

Lesions greater than 4 cm in diameter tend to be metastases or primary adrenal carcinoma.

Increase in lesion size is a useful indicator of malignancy because adenomas are slow to change size. The shape of the adrenal gland can also be helpful in predicting malignancy. Adenomas tend to have smooth margin and homogenous density, whereas metastases or malignant lesion can be heterogeneous and have an irregular shape. But these findings are not specific. The contra-lateral gland may be occasionally atrophic. Most adenomas are homogenous although larger masses may be heterogeneous because of focal areas of necrosis or haemorrhage (Schwartz, 1996).

Currently, intra-cellular lipid content and differences in vascular enhancement patterns of the adrenal mass represent the most specific differences.

Pheochromocytomas

Pheochromocytomas are catecholamime-producing tumors that arise from the paraganglionic cells. Pheochromocytomas originate in the adrenal medulla in 90% of cases. Most extra adrenal pheochromocytomas (paragangliomas) arise in the paravertebral sympathetic ganglia, in the organ of Zuckerkandl (near the aortic bifurcation), rarely in the bladder. 90% occur sporadically, multiple pheochromocytomas occur in 10%, and 10% are malignant.

On unenhanced CT, pheochromocytomas appear as round masses of similar density to surrounding soft tissue, but frequently undergo necrosis so that the mass may have a fluid filled center (Kalra, 2005). Their unenhanced density is almost constantly over ten UH.

The tumors tend to have an average size of 5 cm, calcifications occur in 12%. Pheochromocytomas show intense enhancement following injection of non ionic contrast media (Szolar, 2005).

On MRI, pheochromocytomas are hypointense on T1 weighted images and typically markedly hyperintense on T2 weighed images. Atypical signal intensity on T2 weighted images is seen in 35% of cases.

CT and MRI are equally accurate for identifying adrenal pheochromocytoma. MRI with multi-planar capability has a slight advantage over CT for detecting extra adrenal pheochromocytoma.

On US, pheochromocytomas are well-defined round or ovoid masses with uniform reflectivity but appear heterogeneous when large because of necrosis and haemorrhage.

Accuracy of US is less than CT, MRI and MIBG scintigraphy.

Myelolipomas

Myelolipomas are rare benign tumors composed of myeloid, erythroid and fatty elements, and occasionally calcify.

The imaging appearance is based on the presence of pure mature fat within a lesion.

They appear echogenic at US, with areas of very low attenuation, below – 40HU at CT and hyper intense on T1 weighted sequences. Typically, they become hypo intense on fat-suppressed sequence (Kenney, 1998; Matsuda, 2004).

Adrenal haemorrhage

Adrenal haemorrhage results from trauma, systemic anticoagulation therapy, sepsis or stress.

At unenhanced CT acute adrenal haemorrhage has an increased attenuation of 60 HU.

Adrenal haemorrhage has a typical appearance at MR imaging, depending on the age of the haemorrhage. After contrast media injection there is no enhancement (Kawashima, 1999).

Lymphoma

Lymphoma is unusual and bilateral in most cases and associated with other sites of nodes.

At CT, the mass is homogenous and with soft tissue density that increases slowly and slightly after injection (Glazer, 1983).

Adrenal cysts

Adrenal cysts are rare entities with typical findings at CT and MRI and no enhancement after injection. They appear with low attenuation at CT and thin margins (Tung, 1989).

Tuberculosis, histoplamosis and blastomycosis result in bilateral enlargement of the adrenal gland with fluid-filled appearance, and often calcify.

Metastasis

Metastases of adrenal glands are frequently encountered whether the primary neoplasm is known or not. Most frequent primary neoplasms are in lung, breast, colon, melanoma origin.

Diagnosis relies on CT and MRI showing a unique or bilateral mass containing fluid and haemorrhage, and sometimes calcifications. There is no lipid content and loss of signal on out of phase images is absent. Furthermore, if attenuation can be low at unenhanced CT, washout remains slow and allows differentiation from other adrenal pathology.

If CT and MRI remain ambiguous, 18 FDG PET/CT or adrenal biopsy can be performed if required for staging and prognosis (Yun, 2001).

Conclusion

Certain features can be used with CT or MRI to establish a definitive diagnosis of an adrenal mass. Adrenal carcinomas are rare tumors, usually large and heterogeneous. CT and MRI are necessary for diagnosis and staging. Imaging rules for interpretation must be applied.

CT should be performed after appropriate biochemical screening. If the attenuation of a mass at non enhanced CT is below 10 HU, the mass is a benign adenoma.

If the attenuation is over 10HU, contrast enhanced CT should be performed with delayed acquisition.

An absolute washout of 60% or a relative washout of 40% at 10 minutes (Blake, 2005) indicates an adenoma. If the non hyper functioning mass remains indeterminate at CT, MR imaging followed by resection or adrenal biopsy can be performed if no typical findings are revealed.

References

Bae KT, Fuangtharnthip P, Prasad SR, Joe BN, Heiken JP. Adrenal masses: CT characterization with histogram analysis method. *Radiology* 2003; 228: 735-42.

Blake MA, Sweeney AT, Kalra MK, Maher MM. Collision adrenal tumors on PET/CT. *AJR Am J Roentgenol* 2004; 183: 864-5.

Blake MA, Mannudeep K, Ann T, et al. Distinguishing Bening from Malignant Adrenal Masses: Multi-Detector Row CT Protocol with 10 Minute Delay. *Radiology* 2005; 238: 578-85.

Boland GW, Hahn PF, Pena C, Mueller PR. Adrenal masses: characterization with delayed contrast-enhanced CT. *Radiology* 1997; 202: 693-6.

Boland GW, Lee MJ, Gazelle GS, Halpern EF, McNicholas MM, Mueller PR. Characterization of adrenal masses using unenhanced CT: an analysis of the CT literature. *AJR Am J Roentgenol* 1998; 171: 201-4.

Caoili EM, Korobkin M, Francis IR, Cohan RH, Dunnick NR. Delayed enhanced CT of lipid-poor adrenal adenomas. *AJR Am J Roentgenol* 2000; 175: 1411-5.

Caoili EM, Korobkin M, Francis IR, et al. Adrenal masses: characterization with combined unenhanced and delayed enhanced CT. *Radiology* 2002; 222: 629-33.

Dunnick NR, Korobkin M. Imaging of adrenal incidentalomas: current status. *AJR Am J Roentgenol* 2002; 179: 559-68.

Dunnick NR, Korobkin M, Francis I. Adrenal radiology: distinguishing benign from malignant adrenal masses. *AJR Am J Roentgenol* 1996; 167: 861-7.

Glazer HS, Lee JK, Balfe DM, Mauro MA, Griffith R, Sagel SS. Non-Hodgkin lymphoma: computed tomographic demonstration of unusual extranodal involvement. *Radiology* 1983; 149: 211-7.

Gomez-Rivera F, Medina-Franco H, Arch-Ferrer JE, Heslin MJ. Adrenocortical carcinoma: a single institution experience. *Am Surg* 2005; 71: 90-4.

Gufler H, Eichner G, Grossmann A, et al. Differentiation of adrenal adenomas from metastases with unenhanced computed tomography. *J Comput Assist Tomogr* 2004; 28: 818-22.

Hussain HK, Korobkin M. MR imaging of the adrenal glands. *Magn Reson Imaging Clin N Am* 2004; 12: 515-44.

Israel GM, Korobkin M, Wang C, Hecht EN, Krinsky GA. Comparison of unenhanced CT and chemical shift MRI in evaluating lipid-rich adrenal adenomas. *AJR Am J Roentgenol* 2004; 183: 215-9.

Kalra MK, Blake MA, Boland GW, Hahn PF. CT features of adrenal pheochromocytomas: attenuation value and loss of contrast enhancement. *Radiology* 2005; 236: 1112-3.

Kawashima A, Sandler CM, Ernst RD, et al. Imaging of nontraumatic hemorrhage of the adrenal gland. *Radiographics* 1999; 19: 949-63.

Kawashima A, Sandler CM, Fishman EK, et al. Spectrum of CT findings in nonmalignant disease of the adrenal gland. *Radiographics* 1998; 18: 393-412.

Kenney PJ, Wagner BJ, Rao P, Heffess CS. Myelolipoma: CT and pathologic features. *Radiology* 1998; 208: 87-95.

Korobkin M, Lombardi TJ, Aisen AM, et al. Characterization of adrenal masses with chemical shift and gadolinium-enhanced MR imaging. *Radiology* 1995; 197: 411-8.

Korobkin M, Brodeur FJ, Yutzy GG, et al. Differentiation of adrenal adenomas from nonadenomas using CT attenuation values. *AJR Am J Roentgenol* 1996; 166: 531-6 (a).

Korobkin M, Giordano TJ, Brodeur FJ, et al. Adrenal adenomas: relationship between histologic lipid and CT and MR findings. *Radiology* 1996; 200: 743-7 (b).

Krebs TL, Wagner BJ. MR imaging of the adrenal gland: radiologic-pathologic correlation. *Radiographics* 1998; 18: 1425-40.

Krestin GP, Freidmann G, Fishbach R, Neufang KF, Allolio B. Evaluation of adrenal masses in oncologic patients: dynamic contrast-enhanced MR vs CT. *J Comput Assist Tomogr* 1991; 15: 104-10.

Matsuda T, Abe H, Takase M, et al. Case of combined adrenal cortical adenoma and myelolipoma. *Pathol Int* 2004; 54: 725-9.

Mayo-Smith WW, Lee MJ, McNicholas MM, Hahn PF, Boland GW, Sain S. Characterization of adrenal masses (< 5 cm) by use of chemical shift MR imaging: observer performance versus quantitative measures. *AJR Am J Roentgenol* 1995; 165: 91-5.

McNicholas MM, Lee MJ, Mayo-Smith WW, Hahn PF, Boland GW, Mueller PR. An imaging algorithm for the differential diagnosis of adrenal adenomas and metastases. *AJR Am J Roentgenol* 1995; 165: 1453-9.

Otal P, Escourrou G, Mazerolles C, et al. Imaging features of uncommon adrenal masses with histopathologic correlation. *Radiographics* 1999; 19: 569-81.

Outwater EK, Siegelman ES, Huang AB, Birnbaum BA. Adrenal masses: correlation between CT attenuation value and chemical shift ratio at MR imaging with in-phase and opposed-phase sequences. *Radiology* 1996; 201: 880.

Outwater EK, Siegelman ES, Radecki PD, Piccoli CW, Mitchell DG. Distinction between benign and malignant adrenal masses: value of T1-weighted chemical-shift MR imaging. *AJR Am J Roentgenol* 1995; 165: 579-83.

Paulsen SD, Nghiem HV, Korobkin M, Caoili, EM, Higgins EJ. Changing role of imaging-guided percutaneous biopsy of adrenal masses: evaluation of 50 adrenal biopsies. *AJR Am J Roentgenol* 2004; 182: 1033-7.

Pena CS, Boland GW, Hahn PF, Lee MJ, Mueller PR. Characterization of indeterminate (lipid-poor) adrenal masses: use of washout characteristics at contrast-enhanced CT. *Radiology* 2000; 217: 798-802.

Pommier RF, Brennan, MF. An eleven-year experience with adrenocortical carcinoma. *Surgery* 1992; 112: 963-70; discussion 970-1.

Schwartz LH, Ginsberg MS, Burt ME, Brown KT, Getrajdman GI, Panicek DM. MRI as an alternative to CT-guided biopsy of adrenal masses in patients with lung cancer. *Ann Thorac Surg* 1998; 65: 193-7.

Schwartz LH, Macari M, Huvos AG, Panicek DM. Collision tumors of the adrenal gland: demonstration and characterization at MR imaging. *Radiology* 1996; 201: 757-60.

Schwartz LH, Panicek DM, Koutcher JA, *et al.* Adrenal masses in patients with malignancy: prospective comparison of echo-planar, fast spin-echo, and chemical shift MR imaging. *Radiology* 1995; 197: 421-5.

Silverman SG, Mueller PR, Pinkney LP, Koenker RM, Seltzer SE. Predictive value of image-guided adrenal biopsy: analysis of results of 101 biopsies. *Radiology* 1993; 187: 715-8.

Szolar DH, Kammerhuber F. Quantitative CT evaluation of adrenal gland masses: a step forward in the differentiation between adenomas and nonadenomas? *Radiology* 1997; 202: 517-21.

Szolar DH, Kammerhuber FH. Adrenal adenomas and nonadenomas: assessment of washout at delayed contrast-enhanced CT. *Radiology* 1998; 207: 369-75.

Szolar DH, Korobkin M, Reittner P, *et al.* Adrenocortical carcinomas and adrenal pheochromocytomas: mass and enhancement loss evaluation at delayed contrast-enhanced CT. *Radiology* 2005; 234: 479-85.

Tung GA, Pfister RC, Papanicolaou N, Yoder IC. Adrenal cysts: imaging and percutaneous aspiration. *Radiology* 1989; 173: 107-10.

Yun M, Kim W, Alnafisi N, Lacorte L, Jang S, Alavi A. 18F-FDG PET in characterizing adrenal lesions detected on CT or MRI. *J Nucl Med* 2001; 42: 1795-9.

Chemotherapy for adrenal cortical cancer

François Goldwasser, Xavier Bertagna
Medical Oncology and Endocrine and Metabolic Diseases; Reference Center for Rare Adrenal Gland Diseases; Endocrinology Department, Institut Cochin, INSERM U567, APHP, Cochin Hospital, Faculty of Medicine René Descartes, Univ. Paris 5

Adrenal cortical carcinoma (ACC) remains a disease with very poor prognosis (Luton, 1990; Schteingart, 2005; Allolio 2006). The best probability of cure is when a localized tumor (stage 1 or 2 MacFarlane) can be subjected to complete removal ("curative" surgery). But almost half of the patients are diagnosed at later stages (invasive or metastatic disease) with a survival rate close to 0% at five years for metastatic ACC. Even after "curative surgery" of localized ACC, recurrence occurs in more than 50% of patients.

There is a desperate need for a means of treating advanced ACCs, and possibly also for an adjuvant treatment to prevent recurrence after "curative" surgery of localized ACCs.

The medical management of locally advanced or metastatic ACCs is changing, as is the oncology field in general. In fact, both present treatment and future developments are typical illustrations of the impact of progress in tumor biology in a clinical setting. Until the 90's, the main treatment for metastatic ACCs was o,p'DDD. However, it is difficult to critically appraise the evidence of its efficacy, particularly in early studies that were performed before the routine use of modern imaging techniques. Moreover, o,p'DDD was not always given as a single agent and could be given together with cytotoxic agents. Another limitation is variability of the response criteria for these clinical studies. Additionally, because some of the studies included hormonal improvement as an indicator of clinical response, it has been difficult to document survival advantage, even though a high percentage of remissions were reported.

This Chapter will review the treatment options available today, present the first international randomized trial in metastatic ACC, and suggest some perspectives for future therapeutic options.

Medical treatment of advanced ACC

O,p' DDD: an adrenolytic drug

Historically

In the late 1940s it was found by serendipity that the insecticide DDD induced a selective necrosis of the dog adrenal cortex (Nelson, 1949). A contaminant of the crude DDD preparation exhibited the actual adrenolytic action: 1,1-dichloro-2-(*o*-chlorophenyl)-2-(*p*-chlorophenyl)-ethane or O,p'DDD *(figure 1)*. It was then used in humans in the late 1950s, where it showed an adrenolytic action on ACC (Bergenstal, 1959).

Mode of action

O,p'DDD is a highly lipophilic compound which concentrates in the adrenal glands. There, it provokes mitochondrial degeneration, and the subsequent destruction of the adrenal cortex. It has been proposed that O,p'DDD is actually a pro-drug: in the adrenal it appears to be transformed into an acyl chloride derivative; this latter compound interacts locally with some specific proteins (Cai, 1995).

Kinetic properties

O,p'DDD has particular kinetic properties.

Its absorption rate is very variable, depending on the vehicle. Compared with the commercially available tablets (Lysodren®, HRA-Pharma, France), it is better absorbed when given in milk or chocolate, and less absorbed when micronized into capsules with the gastro-resistant cellulose acetylphtalate (Mitotane, Roussel UCLAF) (Moolenar, 1981): when comparing treatments in the literature one should be aware that, for this reason, Mitotane in capsules was generally given at much higher dose (up to 12g per day) than Lysodren® tablets (up to 6g per day). Lysodren® is now the sole available drug in Europe.

O,p'DDD is stored in the fat, and has been detected in blood as long as 20 months after drug discontinuation.

Side effects

The most common side effects of O,p'DDD are digestive and neurologic. They are somewhat related to the plasma levels of the drug, and rarely occur when plasma O,p'DDD is under 20 mg/L (van Slooten, 1984; Haak, 1994). Nausea, anorexia, vomiting will occur in a majority of patients; apathy, dizziness, ataxia, speech difficulties, lack of concentration and tremor are less frequent. These manifestations are always transient, and disappear after the drug is discontinued for several days. They imply that a fine adjustment of the drug dosage must be obtained, with the help of plasma monitoring.

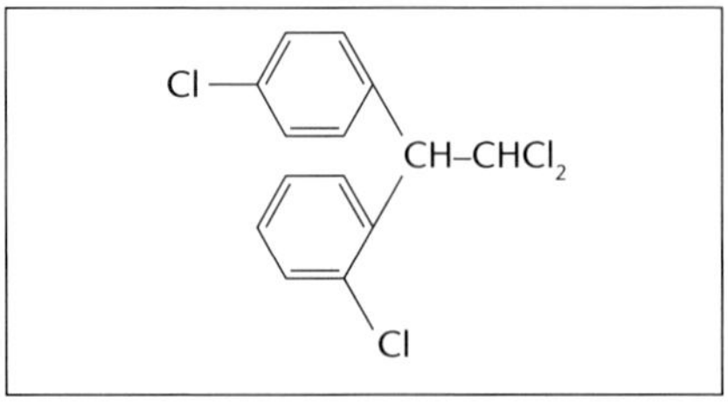

Figure 1. The molecule O,p'DDD.

Because the normal adrenal is also a target of O,p'DDD, adrenal insufficiency is induced in almost all patients. Education, and hormone substitution is necessary, like for Addisonian patients. Since O,p'DDD accelerates liver metabolism of steroids, higher doses of hydrocortisone supplementation are often required. It is wise to eliminate the likelihood of adrenal insufficiency before attributing digestive symptoms to drug intolerance.

O,p'DDD almost always creates a series of biochemical alterations, due to its being an inducer of liver microsomal enzymes: increased liver enzymes, elevated blood cholesterol; caution should be exercised to adjust intercurrent treatment involving liver metabolism (anti-vitamin K, contraceptive pills). Gynecomastia is frequent in males, due to the intrinsic estrogen-like effect of the drug. High increases in plasma CBG and SBG alter the interpretations of plasma cortisol and sex hormones.

Allergic reactions can occur, most often transient; hematologic toxicity is rare (neutropenia). No renal toxicity is reported.

In general, the gonads are not a target for O,p'DDD, although steroidogenesis may be altered, particularly in the testis. Contraception should be insured in the female, since there is evidence for teratogenicity of the drug in humans.

Results of O,p'DDD in advanced ACCs

O,p'DDD was first used in ACC patients by Bergenstal in 1959: he reported on 18 patients, seven of whom showed some tumor regression.

Tumor response to O,p'DDD has since been reported in several series *(figure 2)*:

– Hutter and Kayhoe in 1966 reported a 34% response rate in 59 ACC patients treated with O,p'DDD.

– Luton *et al.* in 1992 observed eight partial tumor regressions out of 37 patients treated.

– In an extensive 1993 review in the English literature, Wooten and King analyzed more than 500 patients who received o,p'DDD: 35% showed a response, which was most often partial and transient.

– Khorram-Manesh *et al.* in 1998 and Baudin *et al.* in 2001 reported somewhat similar response rates of about 30%.

– Analyzing only prospective studies of more than ten patients in the last 20 years, Allolio (2006) found an average response rate of 25%.

An important finding was made when van Slooten in 1984 first reported that proper monitoring of plasma O,p'DDD was instrumental to the follow-up of patients, with two important impacts:

– Plasma O,p'DDD should be under 20 mg/L, to avoid (or minimize!) drug intolerance.

– Plasma O,p'DDD should be over 14 mg/L, to increase the likelihood of tumor response.

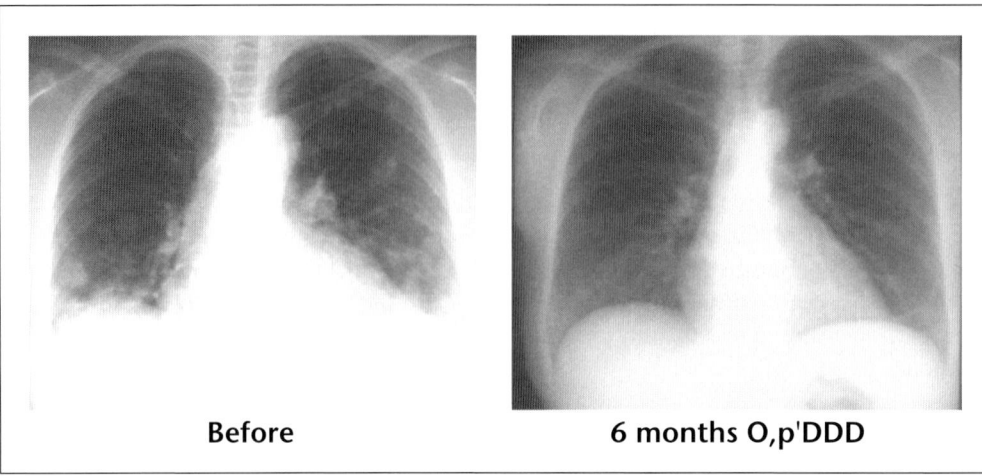

Figure 2. The effect of O,p'DDD treatment on lung metastases.

The usefulness of this indicative range of plasma concentration was confirmed by the consecutive studies of Haak in 1994, and Baudin in 2001.

The role of O, p'DDD on the survival of advanced ACC is not established as well, and is still debated:

– No benefit to survival was found in the retrospective series of 105 patients, conducted by Luton *et al.* in 1992.

– When this series was extended 10 years later to 202 patients (Abiven, 2006), it showed that O,p'DDD had a beneficial effect on survival only in the group of patients with cortisol hypersecretion.

– The study by Icard in 2001 found that O,p'DDD treatment was associated with a longer survival only in patients not oprerated for cure.

Whereas it is clear that all these results were obtained in observational, non-randomized, retrospective series, it is nevertheless agreed that O,p'DDD has an anti tumoral effect in ACC. There is however no proven evidence for a beneficial effect on survival.

Today it seems reasonable to propose O,p'DDD as a first line treatment for advanced ACC, provided that its plasma concentration is tightly monitored to remain in the 14-20 mg/L range, that its tolerance is acceptable, and that close endocrine supervision allows proper substitutive therapy. Approximately one fourth to one third of the patients will show positive tumor response, almost invariably partial and/or transient. In case of failure, or after recurrence, second line cytotoxic chemotherapies should be proposed.

Cytotoxic drugs and regimens

Due to the limited number of patients enrolled in each of the studies in ACC (between 11 and 45 patients included), the confidence intervals of response are wide and overlapping across the different studies.

Cisplatin has been the most widely used drug, either alone or in combination with other agents. However, the management of cisplatin infusions requires careful monitoring since this anticancer agent induces irreversible acute renal toxicity and many ACC patients frequently have a single remaining kidney.

Over the last decade, about 10 prospective studies evaluated the efficacy of various chemotherapy regimens, using standardized criteria for tumor response, in patients with either locally advanced or metastatic ACC (*table I*, from Allolio, 2004). Only one study reported on a single agent experience. In half of the studies, the patients were also given treatment with op'DDD. The rationale for combining op'DDD with cytotoxic agents such as doxorubicin or etoposide is based on the ability of op'DDD to reverse *in vitro* the multidrug resistance phenotype mediated by p-glycoprotein overexpression. This observation, however, was never validated in a clinical setting. The most commonly used combinations were cisplatin-doxorubicin-etoposide.

With the exception of the topoisomerase I poison irinotecan (Baudin *et al.*, 2002), none of the anticancer agents developed after the 90's has been evaluated in this setting to date: gemcitabine, taxanes (docetaxel, paclitaxel). Yet, Paclitaxel was found to have cytotoxic activity *in vitro* against a human adrenocortical carcinoma cell line (Fallo, 1998).

Table I. Cytotoxic chemotherapy studies in ACC.

Cytotoxic agent	Mitotane	n	Complete Response (n)	Partial Response (n)	Total (%)	Reference
D,V,E	+	36	1	4	14	Abraham *et al.*, 2002
S	+	22	1	7	36	Khan *et al.*, 2002
P,E	–	45	0	5	11	Williamson *et al.*, 2000
E,D,P	+	28	2	13	54	Berruti *et al.*, 1998
P,E	+	18	3	3	33	Bonacci *et al.*, 1998
P,E	–	13	0	6	46	Burgess *et al.*, 1993
P	+	37	1	10	30	Bukowski *et al.*, 1993
D	–	16	1	2	19	Decker *et al.*, 1991
D,P,5-FU	–	13	1	2	23	Schlumberger *et al.*, 1991
C,D,P	–	11	0	2	18	van Slooten & van Oosterom, 1983
		239	10	54	27	

D: doxorubicin; E: etoposide; 5-FU: 5-fluorouracil; C: cyclophosphamide; V: vincristine; S: streptozocin; P: cisplatin.
From Allolio B. *et al.*, *Clin Endocrinol* 2004.

To date, the best results were reported in a small series of 28 patients using a combination of low-dose O,p'DDD with etoposide, doxorubicin, and cisplatin (EDP regimen). The overall response rate was 53% including 2 complete responses and 13 partial responses (Berruti, 1998). The same group recently updated these results and reported a response rate of 48.5% and a median survival time of 28 months in a total of 66 patients (Berruti, 2005). The treatment protocol is detailed in *table II*.

Etoposide is a non-intercalator topoisomerase II poison (for recent review: Pommier Y, 2006). Doxorubicin is a DNA intercalant and is also a topoisomerase II poison. Additionally, doxorubicin induced DNA strand breakage mediated by free radicals. Cisplatin induces DNA intra and inter strand crosslinks (Goldwasser F, 1996; Zeghari-Squalli N, 1999). Cisplatin and topoisomerase II poisons are synergistic *in vitro* and in the clinical setting (Pommier Y, 2006). Even though similar interactions were observed when combining cisplatin derivatives with topoisomerase I poisons, the lack of antitumoral activity of the topoisomerase I inhibitor, irinotecan (Baudin E, 2002), did not incite development of platinum-topoisomerase I poison combinations in adrenal cancer patients.

Another group reported on the rather satisfactory response rate (36% complete or partial responses) of a regimen using a combination of streptozotocin and Op'DDD (Khan, 2000); this same group later proposed another combination with vincristine, cisplatin, teniposide, and cyclophosphamide as a second cytotoxic line treatment in case of failure (Khan, 2004).

The FIRM-ACT trial [http//:www.firm-act.org]

In 2003, an International Consensus Meeting on the Treatment of Adrenal Cortical Carcinoma took place at Ann Arbor (Michigan, USA), and its conclusions have been published (Schteingart, 2005). There was general agreement that no satisfactory treatment for ACC was available. It was also apparent that all the data in the international literature were from observational studies, on small series of non-randomized patients.

A proposal was made to launch the first randomized prospective therapeutic trial in ACC, with the prospect to compare the efficacy of two already known drug regimens: these two regimens were chosen on the basis of their putative better efficacies, compared to all others, according to observational studies *(figure 3)*:

– O,p'DDD + streptozotocin, in one arm (Khan, 2000).

– O,p'DDD + cisplatin/etoposide/doxorubicine, in the other arm (Berruti, 1998).

Table II. EDP regimen. Each cycle is repeated every 28 days.

Agent	Daily Dose (mg/m2)	Dose/cycle (mg/m2)	Dose intensity (mg/m2/wk)	Day 1	Day 2	Day 3	Day 4
Doxorubicin	40	40	10	x			
Etoposide	100	300	75		x	x	x
Cisplatin	40	80	20			x	x

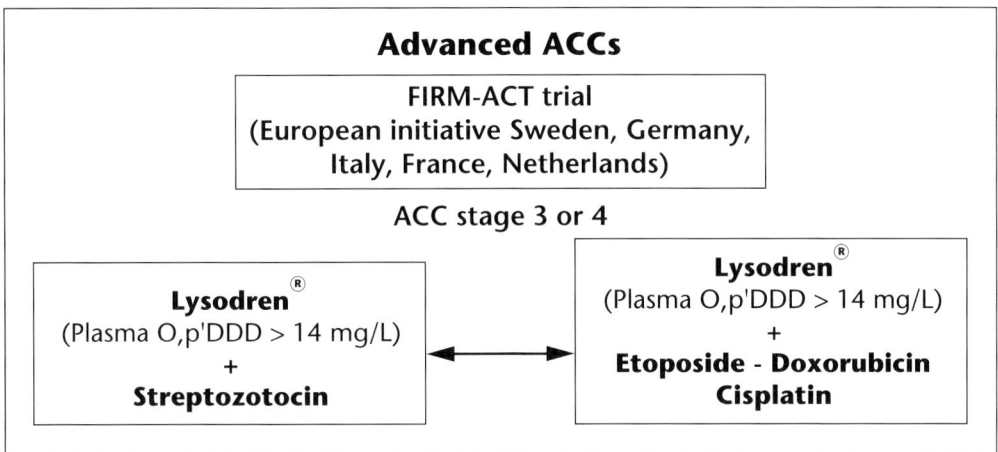

Figure 3. The two arms of the FIRM-ACT Trial.

The trial has been ongoing in Europe for one year. The patients are randomly assigned one treatment, and shifted to the other arm in case of disease progression. Plasma O,p'DDD is closely monitored to insure therapeutic levels.

Adjuvant O,p'DDD treatment after curative surgery?

Because there is a high recurrence rate after "curative" surgery (Luton, 1990), and because O,p'DDD has an antitumoral effect, many authors have empirically used it as an adjuvant therapy, hoping to increase disease-free survival after complete surgery. A survey of the different series reporting on this treatment option is contradictory, with some studies showing some benefit (Venkatesh, 1989; Schteingart, 1982; Dickstein, 1998; Kasperlik-Zaluska, 2000), and others showing no benefit (Luton, 1992; Barzon, 1997; Icard, 2001) or even a detrimental effect (Vassilopoulou-Sellin, 1993). The most recent series, recruiting 102 patients in eight Italian centres, reported in abstract form (Daffara, 2005), seemed more encouraging, showing a strong beneficial effect of Op'DDD in an adjuvant setting: median disease-free survival was 30 months in the adjuvant group versus 10 months in the control group. Yet, this latter series, like all others, was restropective, on non randomized patients.

Thus, there are still no clear answers to the questions: should we systematically treat stage 1 or 2 patients, after complete surgery, with O,p' DDD? Immediately after surgery or even before surgery? For how long? Despite all the side effects of the drug and the induction of adrenal insufficiency, and precluding pregnancy? Should we select patients? On wich prognostic markers?

What is needed today is a prospective randomized trial, to answer these difficult questions. An international effort, again, will be necessary to engage a sufficient number of patients.

Conclusion and perspectives

To date, the medical management of locally advanced or metastatic ACC remains largely frustrating and non curative. As a result, the multidisciplinary discussion is a critical frame to define, on a case by case basis, patients susceptible of benefiting from a potentially curative surgical resection of metastases. Besides surgery, medical treatments are palliative and the gold standard remains O,p'DDD or its addition to a cytotoxic chemotherapy such as the EDP regimen.

Nevertheless, hopes of progress in a clinical setting are not supported by conventional chemotherapy but rather by the rapid development of medical strategies, either based on ACC biology (targeted therapies), or based on the interactions between adrenal cancer cells and their microenvironment (inhibitors of tumor angiogenesis).

The treatment of metastatic cancers is being transformed by targeted therapies (Verweij J. *et al.*, 2003; Cunningham D. *et al.*, 2004) and anti-angiogenic agents (Hurwitz H. *et al.*, 2004). For the first time, the same agent – the monoclonal antibody anti-VEGF, bevacizumab – was found to significantly increase survival in three metastatic cancers as different as breast, lung, and colon cancers. This clinical result is not related to the biology of a given malignant tissue, and thus opens new perspectives for all malignant diseases *(table III)*. As a consequence, it is worthwhile to see whether similar therapies might be of interest in ACC, since overexpression of the VEGF receptor has been demonstrated in ACC (de Fraipont, 2000).

More than 80% of ACCs have a moderate to high intensity for EGF receptors (Kamio, T. *et al.*, 1990). In 62 of 64 patients, there was already metastasis to other organs. The authors concluded that the expression of EGF receptors is associated with tumor growth and/or metastatic potential in adrenocortical carcinoma (Kamio, T. *et al.*, 1990). However, the extent of gene amplification seems a better predictor of the efficacy of anti EGF receptor agents, rather than of its expression (Moroni, M. *et al.* 2005). Therefore, it might be interesting to evaluate the efficacy in a clinical setting of either cetuximab or inhibitors of the tyrosine kinase activity of the EGF receptor, such as erlotinib.

Progress will undoubtedly come from a better understanding of the pathogenesis of adrenal cortex tumorigenesis (Libé, 2005), that will help us to imagine and undertake new therapeutic approaches (Kirschner, 2006). We must trust that the next decade will give us answers concerning the efficacy of these new therapeutic approaches in ACC patients.

Table III. From cancer paradigm to treatment: Applications to adrenal cancer patients.

	1	2	3	4
Cancer is an...	Uncontrolled cell proliferation	Accumulation of somatic mutations	Alterations in signalling pathways and response to stress	Alterations in the cancer cell-environnment crosstalk
Treatment is based on...	Anti-mitotic agent	Cytotoxic polychemotherapy	Targeted therapies	Bisphosphonates, anti-angiogenic agents Metalloproteinase inhibitors
In adrenal cancers	O,p'DDD	EDP regimen	EGF receptor inhibitors?	Anti-angiogenic agents?

References

Abiven G, Coste J, Groussin L, et al. Clinical and biological features in the prognosis of adrenal cortical carcinoma. Poor outcome of cortisol secreting tumors in a series of 202 consecutive patients. *J Clin Endocrinol Metab* 2006; 91: 2650-55.

Ahlman H, Khorram-Manesh A, Jansson S, Wangberg B, Nilsson O, Jacobsson CE, Lindstedt S. Cytotoxic treatment of adrenocortical carcinoma. *World J Surg* 2001; 25: 927-33.

Alexandre J, Gross-Goupil M, Nguyen ML, Gornet JM, Misset JL, Goldwasser F. Evaluation of the nutritional and inflammatory status of cancer patients to assess the risk of severe hematologic toxicity of antineoplastic regimens. *Ann Oncol* 2003; 14 (1): 36-41.

Alexandre J, Nicco C, Chéreau C, Laurent A, Weill B, Goldwasser F, et al. Improvement of the therapeutic index of anticancer drugs by the SOD-mimic mangafodipir. *J Natl Cancer Inst* 2006; 98 (4): 236-44.

Alexandre J, Batteux F, Nicco C, Chereau C, Laurent A, Guillevin L, et al. Accumulation of hydrogen peroxide is an early and crucial step for paclitaxel-induced cancer cell death both in vitro and in vivo. *Int J Cancer* 2006.

Allolio B, Fassnacht M. Adrenocortical Carcinoma: Clinical Update. *J Clin Endocrinol Metab* 2006 Mar 21; [Epub ahead of print].

Allolio B, Hahner S, Weismann D, Fassnacht M. Management of adrenocortical carcinoma. *Clin Endocrinol* 2004; 60: 273-87.

Barzon L, Fallo F, Sonino N, Daniele O, Boscaro M. adrenocortical carcinoma: experience in 45 patients. *Oncology* 1997; 54: 490-6.

Baudin E, Docao C, Gicquel C, Vassal G, Bachelot A, Penfornis A, Schlumberger M. Use of a topoisomerase I inhibitor (irinotecan, CPT-11) in metastatic adrenocortical carcinoma. *Ann Oncol* 2002; 13 (11): 1806-9.

Bergenstal D, Lipsett M, Moy R, Hertz R. Regression of adrenal cancer and suppression of adrenal function in men by O,p'DDD. *Trans Am Phys* 1959; 72: 341.

Berruti A, Terzolo M, Pia A, Angeli A, Dogliotti L. Mitotane associated with etoposide, doxorubicin, and cisplatin in the treatment of advanced adrenocortical carcinoma. *Cancer* 1998; 83: 2194-200.

Berruti A, Terzolo M, Sperone P, Pia A, Casa SD, Gross DJ, Carnaghi C, Casali P, Porpiglia F, Mantero F, Reimondo G, Angeli A, Dogliotti L. Etoposide, doxorubicin and cisplatin plus mitotane in the treatment of advanced adrenocortical carcinoma: a large prospective phase II trial. *Endocr Relat Cancer* 2005; 12 (3): 657-66.

Boven E, Vermorken JB, van Slooten H, Pinedo HM. Complete response of metastasized adrenal cortical carcinoma with o,p'-DDD. Case report and literature review. *Cancer* 1984 Jan 1; 53 (1): 26-9. Review.

Bukowski RM, Wolfe M, Levine HS, Crawford DE, Stephens RL, Gaynor E, Harker WG. Phase II trial of mitotane and cisplatin in patients with adrenal carcinoma: a Southwest Oncology Group study. *J Clin Oncol* 1993; 11 (1): 161-5.

Cai W, Counsell RE, Djanegara T, Schteingart DE, Sinsheimer JE, Wotring LL. Metabolic activation and binding of mitotane in adrenal cortex homogenates. *J Pharm Sci* 1995; 84 (2): 134-8.

Cunningham D, Humblet Y, Siena S, et al. Cetuximab monotherapy and cetuximab plus irinotecan in irinotecan-refractory metastatic colorectal cancer. *N Engl J Med* 2004; 351 (4): 337-45.

Daffara F, Reimondo G, Conton P, et al. Adjuvant Mitotane therapy in patients with adrenal cortical carcinoma. European Congress of Endocrinology, Goteborg, September 2005.

Days RS. Treatment sequencing, asymmetry, and uncertainty: protocol strategies for combination chemotherapy. *Cancer Res* 1986; 46: 3876-85.

De Fraipont F, El Atifi M, Gicquel C, Bertagna X, Chambaz EM, Feige JJ. Expression of the angiogenesis markers VEGF-A, thrombospondi-1, and platelet-derived endothelial cell growth in human sporadic adrenocortical tumors: correlation with genotyping alteration. *J Clin Endocrinol Metab* 2000; 85: 4734-41.

Dickstein G, Shechner C, Arad E, Best LA, Nativ O. Is there a role for low doses of mitotane (o,p'-DDD) as adjuvant therapy in adrenocortical carcinoma? *J Clin Endocrinol Metab* 1998; 83 (9): 3100-3.

Fallo F, Pilon C, Barzon L, et al. Paclitaxel is an effective antiproliferative agent on the human NCI-H295 adrenocortical carcinoma cell line. *Chemotherapy* 1998; 44 (2): 129-34.

Goldwasser F, Bae I, Valenti M, Torres K, Pommier Y. Topoisomerase I-related parameters and camptothecin activity in the colon carcinoma cell lines from the NCI anticancer screen. *Cancer Res* 1995; 55: 2116-21.

Goldwasser F, Shimizu T, Jackman J, et al. Correlations between S- and G2-phase arrest and the cytotoxicity of camptothecin in human colon carcinoma cells. *Cancer Res* 1996; 56: 4430-76.

Goldwasser F, Valenti M, Torres R, Pommier Y. Potentiation of cisplatin cytotoxicity by 9-aminocamptothecin. *Clin Cancer Res* 1996; 2: 687-93.

Goldwasser F, Bozec L, Zéghari-Squalli N, Jean-Louis Misset. Cellular pharmacology of the combination of oxaliplatin with topotecan in the IGROV1 human ovarian cancer cell line. *Anti-Cancer Drugs* 1999; 10 (2): 195-201.

Goldwasser F, Gross-Goupil M, Tigaud JM, et al. Dose escalation of CPT-11 in combination with oxaliplatin using an every two weeks schedule: a phase I study in advanced gastrointestinal cancer patients. *Ann Oncol* 2000; 11: 1463-70.

Haak HR, Hermans J, van de Velde CJ, Lentjes EG, Goslings BM, Fleuren GJ, Krans HM. Optimal treatment of adrenocortical carcinoma with mitotane: results in a consecutive series of 96 patients. *Br J Cancer* 1994; 69 (5): 947-51.

Hahner S, Fassnacht M. Mitotane for adrenocortical carcinoma treatment. *Curr Opin Investig Drugs* 2005; 6 (4): 386-94. Review.

Hurwitz H, Fehrenbacher L, Novotny W, et al. Bevacizumab plus irinotecan, fluorouracil, and leucovorin for metastatic colorectal cancer. *N Engl J Med* 2004; 350 (23): 2335-42.

Hutter AM, Kayhoe DE. Adrenal cortical carcinoma. Results of treatment with o,p'DDD in 138 patients. *Am J Med* 1966; 41: 581-92.

Icard P, Goudet P, Charpenay C, Andreassian B, Carnaille B, Chapuis Y, Cougard P, Henry JF, Proye C. Adrenocortical carcinomas: surgical trends and results of a 253-patient series from the French Association of Endocrine Surgeons study group. *World J Surg* 2001; 25: 891-7.

Kamio T, Shigematsu K, Sou H, Kawai K, Tsuchiyama H. Immunohistochemical expression of epidermal growth factor receptors in human adrenocortical carcinoma. *Hum Pathol* 1990; 21 (3): 277-82.

Kasperlik-Zaluska AA. Clinical results of the use of mitotane for adrenal cortical carcinoma. *Braz J Med Biol Res* 2000; 33: 1191-6.

Khan TS, Imam H, Juhlin C, Skogseid B, Grondal S, Tibblin S, Wilander E, Oberg K, Eriksson B. Streptozocin and o,p'DDD in the treatment of adrenal cortical carcinoma patients: long-term survival in its adjuvant use. *Ann Oncol* 2000; 11 (10): 1281-7.

Khan TS, Sundin A, Juhlin C, Wilander E, Oberg K, Eriksson B. Vincristine, cisplatin, teniposide, and cyclophosphamide combination in the treatment of recurrent or metastatic adrenal cortical carcinoma. *Med Oncol* 2004; 21 (2): 167-77.

Kirschner LS. Emerging treatment strategies for adrenocortical carcinoma: a new hope. *J Clin Endocrinol Metab* 2006; 91 (1): 14-21. Epub 2005 Oct 18. Review.

Laurent A, Nicco C, Chéreau C, Goulvestre C, Alexandre J, Alves A, *et al*. Controlling tumor growth by modulating endogenous production of reactive oxygen species. *Cancer Res* 2005; 65 (3): 948-56.

Libé R, Bertherat J. Molecular genetics of adrenocortical tumors, from familial to sporadic diseases. *Eur J Endocrinol* 2005; 153 (4): 477-87. Review.

Luton JP, Cerdas S, Billaud L, Thomas G, Guilhaume B, Bertagna X, Laudat MH, Louvel A, Chapuis Y, Blondeau P, *et al*. Clinical features of adrenocortical carcinoma, prognostic factors, and the effect of mitotane therapy. *N Engl J Med* 1990; 322: 1195-201.

Moolenar AJ, Van Slooten H, Van Seters AP, Smeenk D. Blood levels of O,p'DDD following administration in various vehicles after a single dose and during long term treatment. *Cancer Chemother Pharmacol* 1981; 7: 51-4.

Moroni M, Veronese S, Benvenuti S, Marrapese G, Sartore-Bianchi A, Di Nicolantonio F, Gambacorta M, Siena S, Bardelli A. Gene copy number for epidermal growth factor receptor (EGFR) and clinical response to antiEGFR treatment in colorectal cancer: a cohort study. *Lancet Oncol* 2005; 6 (5): 279-86.

Nelson AA, Woodard G. Severe adrenal cortical atrophy (cytotoxic) and hepatic damage produced in dogs by feeding 2,2-bis- (parachlorophenyl)-1,1-dichloroethane (DDD). *Arch Pathol* 1949; 48: 387.

Norton L, Simon R. Tumor size, sensitivity to therapy and the design of treatment schedules. *Cancer Treat Rep* 1977; 61: 1307-17.

Pommier Y, Goldwasser F. Topoisomerase II inhibitors: The Epipodophyllotoxins, Acridines, and Ellipticines. In: *Cancer Chemotherapy & Biotherapy. Principles and Practice. Chap 19: 451-475*. Chabner B.A. and Longo DL. Ed. J.B. Lippincott Company. 4th Edition 2006.

Schteingart DE, Motazedi A, Noonan RA, Thompson NW. Treatment of adrenal carcinomas. *Arch Surg* 1982; 117: 1142-6.

Schteingart DE, Doherty GM, Gauger PG, Giordano TJ, Hammer GD, Korobkin M, Worden FP. Management of patients with adrenal cancer: recommendations of an international consensus conference. *Endocr Relat Cancer* 2005; 12 (3): 667-80. Review.

van Slooten H, Moolenaar AJ, van Seters AP, Smeenk D. The treatment of adrenocortical carcinoma with o,p'-DDD: prognostic implications of serum level monitoring. *Eur J Cancer Clin Oncol* 1984; 20 (1): 47-53.

Vassilopoulouu-Sellin R, Guinee VF, klein MJ, Taylor SH, Hess KR, Schultz PN, Samaan NA. Impact of adjuvant Mitotane on the clinical course of patients with adrenal cortical carcinoma. *Cancer* 71: 3119-23.

Venkatesh S, Hickey RC, Sellin RV, Fernandez JF, Samaan NA. Adrenal cortical carcinoma. *Cancer* 1989 Aug 1; 64 (3): 765-9.

Verweij J, Casali PG, Zalcberg J, LeCesne A, Reichardt P, Blay JY, Issels R, van Oosterom A, Hogendoorn PC, Van Glabbeke M, Bertulli R, Judson I. Progression-free survival in gastrointestinal stromal tumors with high-dose imatinib: randomised trial. *Lancet* 2004; 364 (9440): 1127-34.

Williamson SK, Lew D, Miller GJ, Balcerzak SP, Baker LH, Crawford ED. Phase II evaluation of cisplatin and etoposide followed by mitotane at disease progression in patients with locally advanced or metastatic adrenocortical carcinoma: a Southwest Oncology Group Study. *Cancer* 2000; 88 (5): 1159-65.

Wooten MD, King DK. Adrenal cortical carcinoma. Epidemiology and treatment with mitotane and a review of the literature. *Cancer* 1993; 72: 3145-55.

Zeghari-Squalli N, Raymond E, Cvitkovic E, Goldwasser F. Cellular pharmacology of the combination of the DNA topoisomerase I inhibitor SN-38 with the Diaminocyclohexane platinum derivative oxaliplatin. *Clin Cancer Res* 1999; 5: 1189-96.

Surgical treatment of adrenal cortical carcinoma

Bertrand Dousset, Sébastien Gaujoux, Jean-Marc Thillois
Department of Digestive and Endocrine Surgery, Cochin Hospital, Paris, Univ. Paris 5, APHP

Introduction

Primary adrenal cortical carcinoma is a rare endocrine tumor with a reported incidence of 0.5 to 2 cases per million (Third National Cancer Survey, 1975; Crucitti, 1996; Dackiw, 2001) leading to 0.1 to 0.2% of cancer deaths (Wajchenberg, 2000). It is one of the most malignant endocrine tumor, with 20 to 40% of synchronous metastatic disease at the time of diagnosis (Abiven, 2006; Icard, 1992a; Venkatesh, 1989) which are mainly located in the liver (44-93%), the lungs (46-79%) and less frequently in the bones (7-24%) (Abiven, 2006; Icard, 1992a; King, 1979; Luton, 1990). The 5-year overall survival is poor ranging from 30 to 40% in most series (Icard, 1992a; Icard, 1992b; Vassilopoulou-Sellin, 2001; Venkatesh, 1989). The prognosis of primary adrenal cortical carcinoma is depending on the stage of the tumor according to the classification of MacFarlane and Sullivan (Sullivan, 1978) *(table I)*. It is also influenced by the semi-quantitative histopronostic score of Weiss (Aubert, 2002; Weiss, 1984) based on presence or absence of the following nine histologic features: high mitotic rate, atypical mitoses, high nuclear grade, low percentage of clear cells, necrosis, diffuse tumor architecture, capsular invasion, sinusoidal invasion and venous invasion *(table II)*. Complete surgical resection is the only potential of cure. There is however some debate regarding the extent of resection, the best surgical approach, the benefits of resection of the primary in case of metastatic disease, the indication of agressive resection for recurrent adrenal cortical carcinoma and resectable metastatic disease.

Locally-advanced adrenal cortical carcinomas, which include MacFarlane stage III and IV tumors with either locoregional or metastatic spread, represent a challenging surgery to achieve complete R0 resection while minimizing both surgical complications and mortality. In this setting, complete removal of the tumor often requires technical constraints depending on the size of the tumor and type of locoregional or metastatic spread: large abdominal or thoraco-abdominal approach, "en-bloc" resection with primary vascular control, lymphadenectomy, ipsilateral nephrectomy, caval thrombectomy with or without caval reconstruction, "en-bloc" resection of adjacent organs, combined hepatectomy or radiofrequency thermoablation of small-size liver metastases.

Table I. Classification of MacFarlane-Sullivan.

Stage	Classification of MacFarlane-Sullivan
I	Tumor < 5 cm, N0, M0
II	Tumor > 5 cm, N0, M0
III	Tumor with locoregional involvement, N0, M0 or Tumor without locoregional involvement, N1, M0
IV	Tumor with locoregional involvement, N1, M0 Or any Tumor, Nx, M1

Table II. Histologic criteria of Weiss score (0 to 9): a score equal to or higher than 3 is indicative of malignancy.

Histologic criteria	Semi-quantitative criteria	Calculation of score
High mitotic rate	> 5/50 High-power fields	0 or 1
Atypical mitoses	Present or absent	0 or 1
High nuclear grade	Present or absent	0 or 1
Low percentage of clear cells	< 25% of tumor cells	0 or 1
Foci of confluent necrosis	Present or absent	0 or 1
Diffuse architectural pattern	> 33% of tumor	0 or 1
Venous invasion	Present or absent	0 or 1
Sinusoidal invasion	Present or absent	or 1
Capsular invasion	Present or absent	0 or 1

Clinical presentation of primary adrenal cortical carcinoma

Epidemiologic data and clinical features of adrenal cortical carcinoma are summarized in *table III*. In brief, primary adrenal cortical carcinoma is arising slightly more frequently in women (Abiven, 2006; Wooten, 1993). According to principal single-center series or national surgical registries, stage I and II disease represent 33 to 56% of the cases, stage III and IV 44 to 77% of the cases (Crucitti, 1996; Harrison, 1999; Icard, 2001; Vassilopoulou-Sellin, 2001; personal data). Primary adrenal cortical carcinoma is similarly affecting the right and left adrenal, at a mean age varying between 46 and 53 years. The prevalence of hormonal hypersecretion is ranging from 34 to 73%, whereas reported means of weight and size at pathologic examination of surgical specimen ranged between 689-764 g and 12-15 cm, respectively (Crucitti, 1996; Harrison, 1999; Icard, 2001; Vassilopoulou-Sellin, 2001; personal data). The presentation of primary ACC may vary with three main clinical patterns.

Table III. Clinical features of primary adreno cortical carcinoma according to principal series.

Centre	N cases (study period)	Gender (F/M)	Stage I-II/ III-IV	Secreting/non secreting	Side R/L	Mean weight (g)	Mean size (cm)
MD Anderson (Vassilopoulou-Sellin, 2001)	139 (1980-2000)	60/40%	33/77%	34/66%	44/56%	–	12
French registry (Icard, 2001)	253 (1978-1997)	62/38%	56/44%	66/34%	–	689	12
Italian registry (Crucitti, 1996)	129 (1980-1995)	58/42%	49/51%	46/54%	50/50%	–	–
Mayo Clinic (Kendrick, 2001)	58 (1980-1996)	48/52%	52/48%	47/53%	53/47%	604	12.5
Memorial Sloan-Kettering (Harrison, 1999)	46 (1986-1996)	65/35%	–	–	48/52%	–	15
Cochin surgical series (personal data)	104 (1980-2002)	75/25%	45/55%	73/27%	52/48%	764	12.8

Overt clinical syndrome of hormonal hypersecretion

According to the literature *(table IV)*, overt clinical syndrome of hormonal hypersecretion is the most frequent clinical presentation of primary ACC, representing 46 to 56% of the cases. The syndrome consists of mixed hypersecretion of cortisol and androgens (47% of secreting tumors), pure hypercortisolism (Cushing's syndrome) (27%), pure virilization (6%) due to androgen hypersecretion or various combinations of steroid oversecretion (20%) (Abiven, 2006). Aldosterone, estradiol and steroid precursors secreting tumors are less frequent. Even though an overt clinical syndrome of hormonal oversecretion is present in half of the cases, a thorough hormonal workup in patients with primary ACC is likely to demonstrate an abnormal secretion in up to 75% of the patients (Abiven, 2006). Thus, overall, 67% of our patients presented cortisol oversecretion, 48% presented androgen oversecretion, 10% presented aldosterone oversecretion, 3% present estradiol oversecretion and 3% had an excess of steroid precursors (Abiven, 2006).

Symptomatic abdominal mass

Nearly 30% of patients with primary ACC present with a mass syndrome. This may include abdominal or dorsal pain, a palpable mass, weight loss, fever of unknown origin, signs of inferior vena cava compression, signs of left-sided portal hypertension (Pommier, 1992). Despite frequent huge tumors, complications such as tumor rupture or haemorrhage are rarely encountered (Crucitti, 1996; Icard, 2001, personal data).

Table IV. Clinical presentation of primary adreno cortical carcinoma according to principal series.

Centre	Symptomatic mass	Signs of hormonal secretion	Incidentaloma
French registry (Icard, 2001)	38%	56%	6%
Italian registry (Crucitti, 1996)	44%	46%	10%
Cochin surgical series (personal data)	35%	56%	9%

Adrenal incidentaloma

The diagnosis of primary ACC is more rarely made (10%) after complete hormonal and imaging work-up in patients presenting with an adrenal incidentaloma. To our knowledge, the smallest metastasizing adrenal cortical carcinoma first reported by our group, was 3 cm in size and weighed 25 g (Gicquel, 1994b). The size of the adrenal mass, as measured on computed tomography (CT) or magnetic resonance imaging (MRI) remains the single best indicator of malignancy (Dackiw, 2001; Ross, 1990). In a retrospective multi-institutional review of incidentalomas, Terzolo et al. reported that a size of 5 cm or more had a sensitivity of 93% and a specificity of 64% for identifying adrenal cortical carcinoma (Terzolo, 1997). For smaller incidentalomas 3 to 5 cm in diameter, CT and MRI criteria for malignancy assume increased importance with respect to surgical indication. Like others, it has been our policy to recommend adrenalectomy for incidentalomas greater than 4 cm in diameter in patients without severe comorbid disease, secreting incidentalomas regardless of tumor size, those with suspicious imaging characteristics regardless of tumor size, or any tumor with objective increase in size during follow-up. Besides the size, the question remains whether a presumably benign adrenocortical adenoma may turn into a malignant tumor with time. There is convincing evidence that adrenal cortical carcinomas are monoclonal whereas the majority of adrenal adenomas displayed patterns of polyclonality (Gicquel, 1994b). Conversely, genetic alterations including loss of heterozygosity at the 17p13 and 11p15 loci and overexpression of the insulin-like growth factor II (IGF-II) gene are associated with the malignant phenotype in sporadic adrenocortical tumors and very rarely seen in adenomas (Gicquel, 1994a; Gicquel, 2000; Gicquel, 1997). We recently observed a focus of true adrenal cortical carcinoma within a 6-cm benign adrenal adenoma in a 62-year old patient, indicating that a benign adenoma may potentially turn into malignancy. Further studies are needed to establish whether subsets of adrenal adenomas are likely to malignant changes over time.

Preoperative evaluation

The preoperative evaluation includes clinical examination, complete biochemical and hormonal assessment, imaging work-up in order to precise the stage and resectability of the tumor, the need for "en-bloc" resection of adjacent organs, the secreting pattern (if any) of the tumor.

Clinical examination

As mentioned above, physical examination will pay particular attention to a huge palpable mass, signs of hormonal overseretion (Cushing's syndrome, virilization), and signs of compression: inferior vena cava compression with related risks of venous thrombosis for right ACC, left-sided portal hypertension for left ACC. The percentage of weight loss, the performance status, a past history of abdominal surgery and the research of comorbid disease are additional important issues with respect to surgical risks.

Biochemical and hormonal measurements

Conventional biochemistry is of particular importance before potential major surgery to screen for biological abnormalities, especially in the setting of primary ACC: hyperglycemia (hypercortisolism), hypokaliema (mineralocorticoid excess), low serum albumin level or impaired hemostasis (denutrition), low hemoglobin level (inflammatory response, portal hypertension), low platelet count (hypersplenism secondary to portal hypertension), creatininemia. In case of abnormal renal function, the measurement of creatinin clearance and renal scintigraphy before ipsilateral nephrectomy may be helpful.

Complete hormonal work-up is mandatory including both the cortical and the medullary adrenal functions to assess the profile of oversecretion and rule out a pheochromocytoma.

Imaging studies

The baseline imaging work-up to assess both loco-regional invasion and metastatic spread of primary ACC includes thoraco-abdominal CT scan, abdominal MRI and ^{18}FDG-PET scan. In case of inferior cava compression or intracaval thrombus extension, venous and caval doppler ultrasound, trans-esophageal echocardiography and angio-MRI with caval reconstruction are also performed. As required by the clinical situation (comorbid disease), lung function tests and echocardiography may be also required. We routinely perform a preoperative venous doppler ultrasound to rule out a silent deep venous thrombosis, especially in the setting of bulky primary tumor or estrogen- or cortisol-hypersecreting tumor.

Predicting malignancy of an adrenal mass

Clinical and biochemical factors suggestive of malignancy

Even though non specific, the presence of a huge palpable mass responsible for abdominal pain is highly suggestive of malignant tumor, especially in the setting of inferior vena cava compression. Biochemically, the presence of a combined hormonal secretion (cortisol and androgens), the presence of a virilization (androgens) or feminizing (estradiol) syndrome, or the oversecretion of inactive steroid precursors are specifically observed in primary ACC.

Imaging characteristics of malignant adrenal lesions

CT scan

On CT scan, typical features of primary adrenal cortical carcinoma are those of a large adrenal mass, greater than 6 cm, poorly delineated, with areas of necrosis and inhomogeneous enhancement following contrast injection, which may contains calcifications secondary to intra-tumoral hemorrhage. The presence of enlarged aorto-caval lymph nodes, local invasion to adjacent organs, intracaval partial or obstructive tumor thrombus, or metastatic hepatic spread are highly suggestive of malignant adrenal tumor *(figures 1, 2 and 3)*.

For smaller adrenal lesions 3 to 6 cm in diameter, CT scan criteria for malignancy have been established, provided helical CT scan with thin slices is performed under specific conditions: CT scan with measurement of spontaneous density (without injection) of the adrenal tumor and repeat measurement of density immediately and 15 minutes after contrast injection, the ratio of which giving the percentage of washout. Several radiological studies have demonstrated that most malignant lesions show a density greater than 20 Hounsfields Units (HU) with a washout less than 50% after a 15 min delay (Boland, 1998; Korobkin, 1998). The specificity of these criteria, in addition to MRI findings is more than 90% to exclude benign adenoma and justify surgical resection.

Magnetic Resonance imaging

On MRI, primary ACC appears hypo or isointense relative to the liver on T1-weighted images with inhomogeneous enhancement following gadolinium injection and hyper- or isointense on T2-weighted images. The patterns of MRI findings are consistent with those of CT scan regarding size, lymph node involvement, locoregional involvement, inferior vena caval invasion and metastatic spread *(figures 1 and 3)*. With the advent of dynamic gadolinium enhanced and chemical shift techniques, MRI has become a reliable method for the differentiation of adenomas from non-adenomas with sensitivies and specificities ranging between 85 and 100% in recently published series (Honigschnabl, 2002; Prager, 2002). Korobkin (1996) and Outwater (1996) showed that the presence of lipids in adrenal adenomas accounted for the low attenuation on unhanced CT, causing a substantial loss of signal intensity on chemical shift MR imaging.

For smaller adrenal lesions 3 to 6 cm in diameter, MRI criteria for malignancy include strong enhancement after gadolinium injection on T1-weighted sequences with delayed post-contrast washout similar to that observed on post-contrast CT-scan, and weak loss of signal intensity on opposed-phase images when compared to in-phase images (Korobkin, 1996; Outwater, 1996; Prager, 2002).

Positron Emission Tomography (PET-scan)

The most frequently used tracer for PET-scan is 18F-fluoro-2deoxy-D-glucose (^{18}FDG). The increased glycolytic metabolism in most malignant tumors accounts for an increase uptake of radiolabeled FDG. Pilot prospective studies have reported PET scan to be highly sensitive (95-100%)

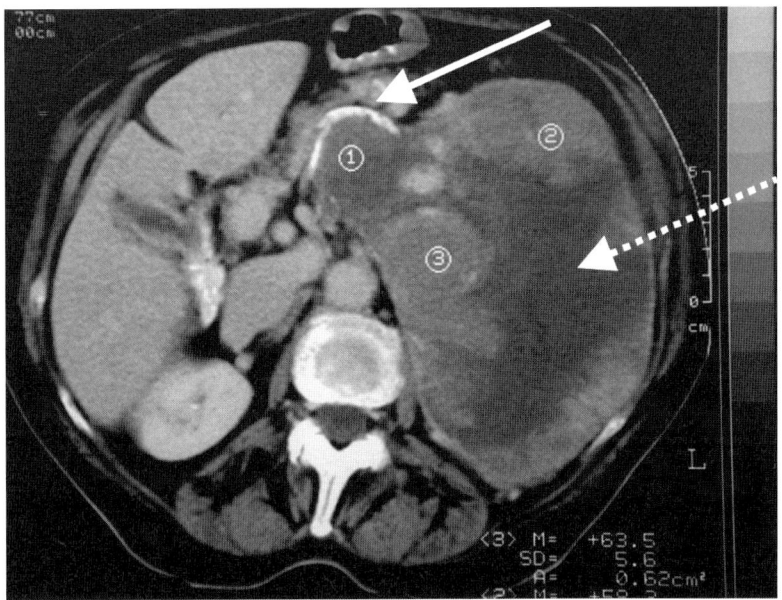

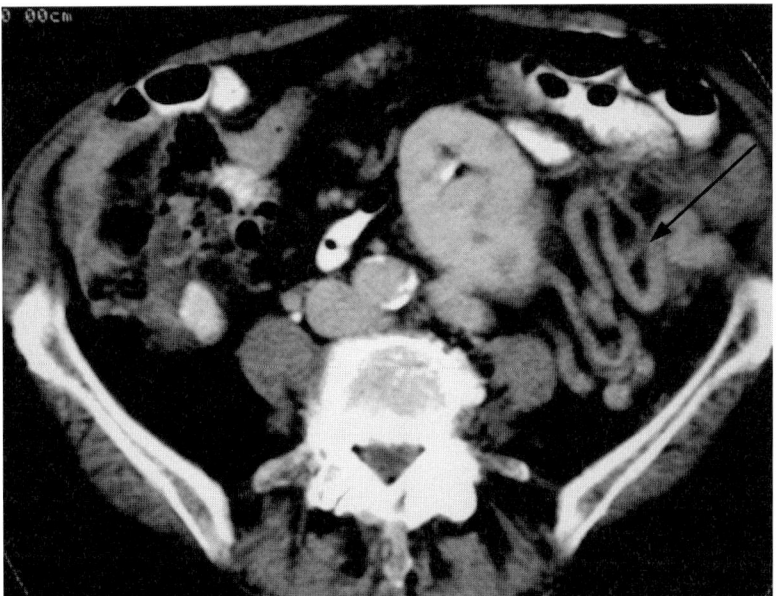

Figure 1a. Left adrenal cortical carcinoma with left-sided portal hypertension. CT scan findings.
White arrow: peripheral calcifications and free dissection plane behind the pancreas.
White dotted arrow: large areas of necrosis with inhomogenous enhancement following contrast injection.
Black arrow: spontaneous splenorenal portasystemic shunt due to left-sided portal hypertension.

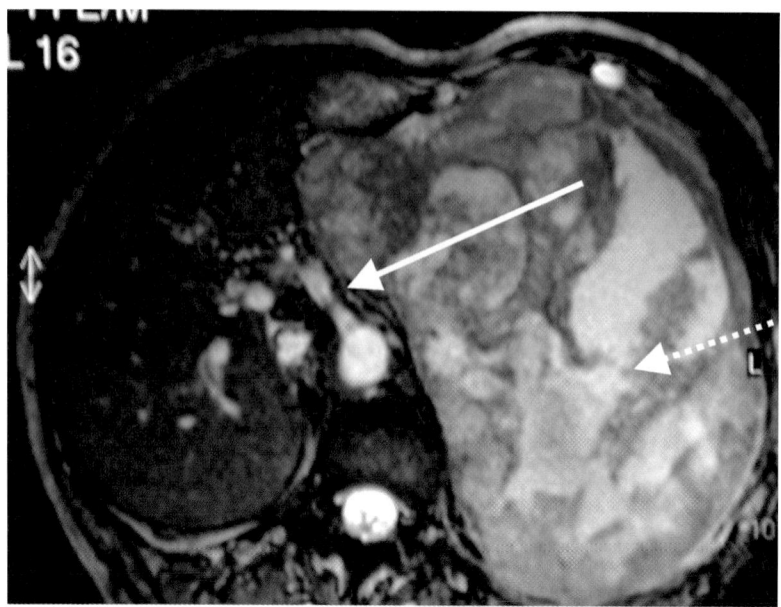

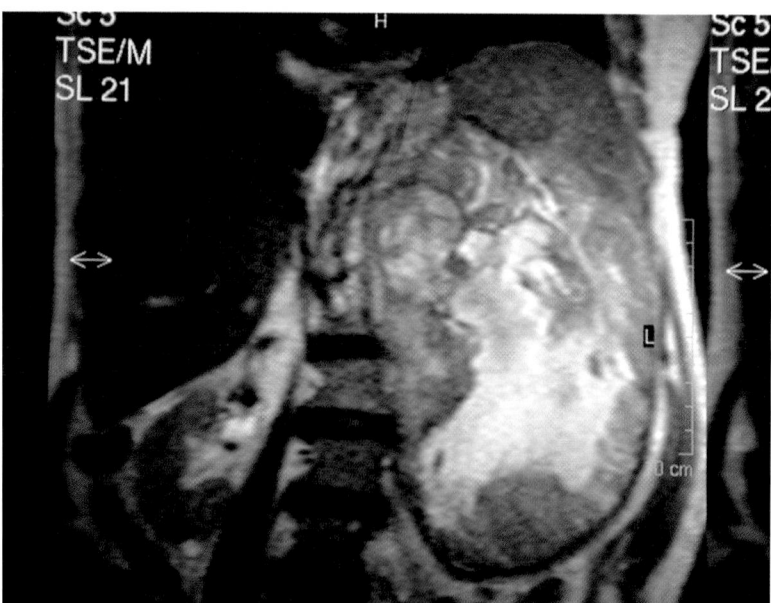

Figure 1b. Left adrenal cortical carcinoma with left-sided portal hypertension. MRI findings
White arrow: right deviation of the celiac axis.
White dotted arrow: larges areas of necrosis with inhomogenous enhancement following gadolinium injection on T1-weighted sequences.
Coronal reconstruction demonstrating medial preaortic extension of left ACC.

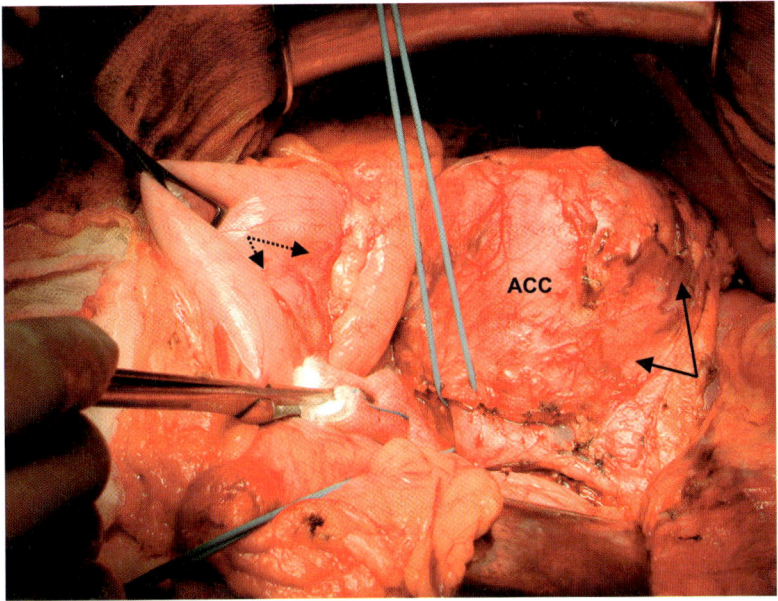

Figure 1c. Operative view of the same patient. Left adrenal vein and left renal vein are retracted by blue silastic tapes. Surgical resection included left adrenal tumor and left kidney. See abnormal feeding vessels (black arrows) and left-sided portal hypertension (dotted black arrows).

and specific (91-94%) in differentiating benign from malignant adrenal tumors (Becherer, 2001; Tenenbaum, 2004). Furthermore, it may play an important role for the diagnosis of metastatic adrenal disease missed by conventional imaging studies. Further studies currently in process are needed to assess the diagnostic accuracy of PET scan for the diagnosis of primary ACC *(figure 4)*.

Surgical indications and preoperative treatment

Primary adrenal cortical carcinomas are staged according to the classification described by MacFarlane and modified by Sullivan. All patients with stage I, II or III disease should be offered surgical resection. Indications for surgery in patients with stage IV disease are more debatable, since median survival time is about 5 months and one-year survival rate is 15%. The decision should take into account the control of symptoms (mass syndrome or hormonal oversecretion) by medical therapy, the age of the patient, the presence of cormorbid disease, and the spread of metastatic disease. Solitary or less than 3 hepatic resectable metastases should not per se contraindicate surgical resection, in view of potential increased survival, quality of palliation and safety of surgery in experienced hands. Similarly, patients with primary ACC extending into the inferior vena cava, which represented 14% in our series, are exposed to severe risks of pulmonary embolism and should be considered for surgery, despite metastatic disease present in half of the cases (Chiche, 2006).

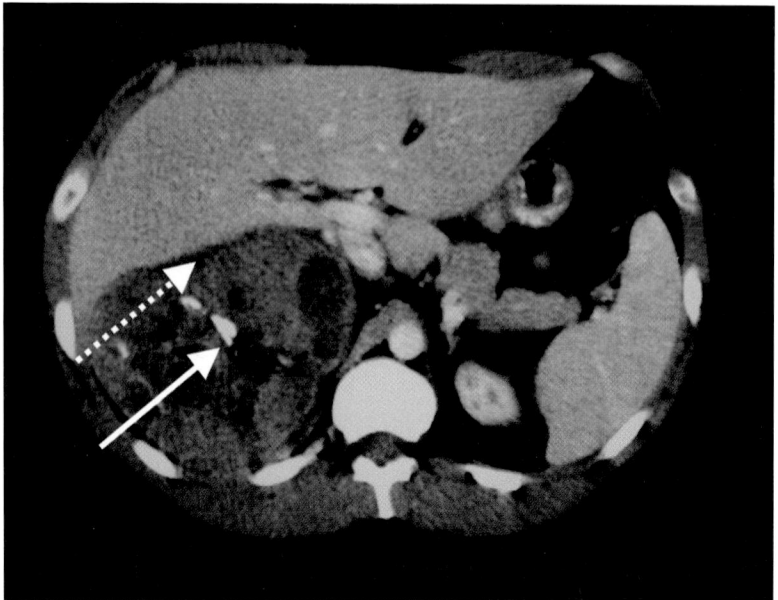

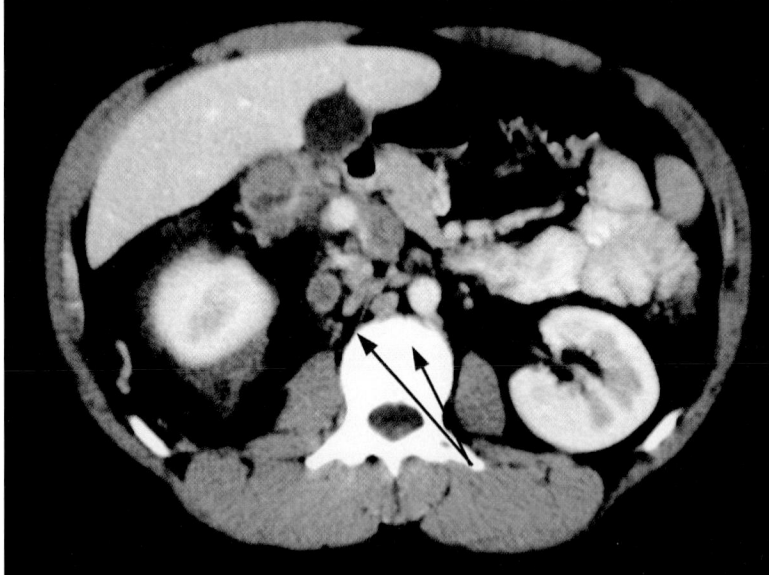

Figure 2. Right adrenal cortical carcinoma with lymph node invasion.
CT scan findings.
White arrow: intratumoral calcifications.
White dotted arrow: clear dissection plane with the liver.
Black arrows: enlarged metastatic lymph nodes.

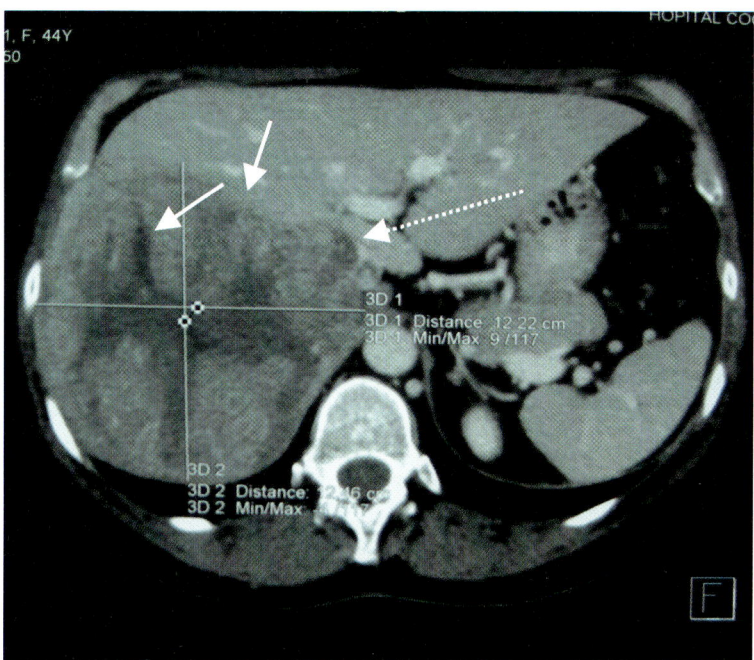

Figure 3. Right adrenal cortical carcinoma with contiguous invasion to the liver and vena caval invasion. CT scan and MRI findings.
White arrows: invasion of adjacent liver.
White dotted arrows: Intracaval invasion with tumoral thrombus.
Figure 3a. CT scan.

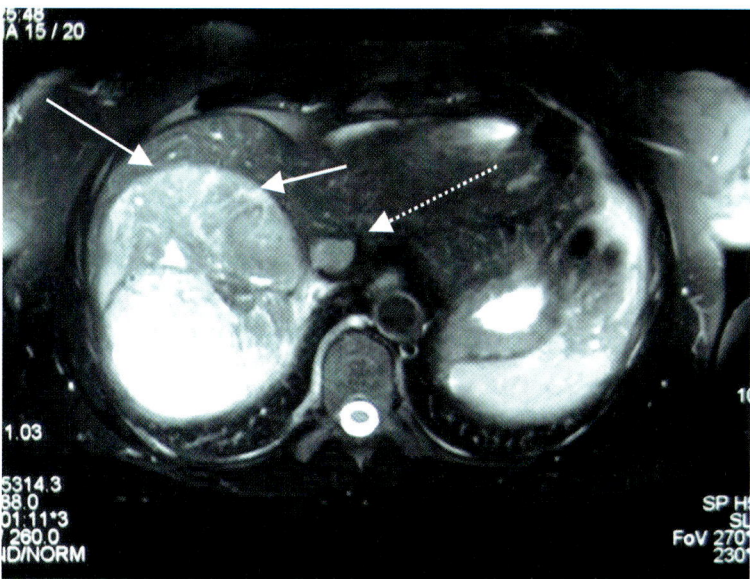

Figure 3b. MRI.

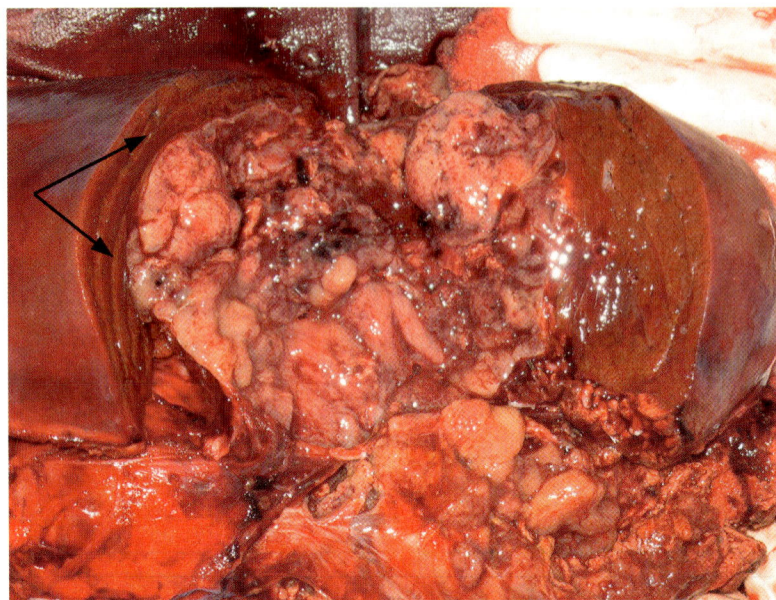

Figure 3c. Macroscopic view of surgical specimen: see massive invasion of hepatic parenchyma (black arrows).

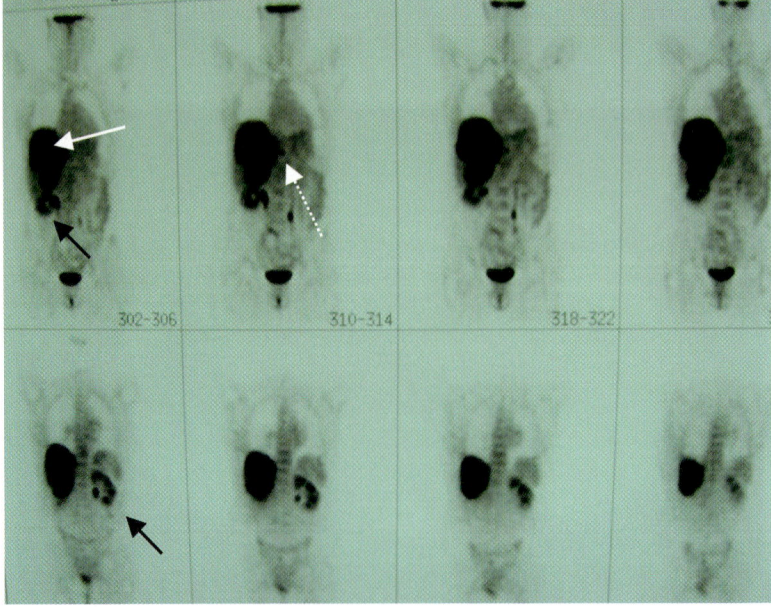

Figure 4. PET scan images of a right adrenocortical carcinoma with increased uptake of the tumor.
Black arrows: right and left kidneys.
White arrow: massive increased uptake of the right ACC with hepatic invasion.
Dotted white arrow: separate area of increased uptake corresponding to a celiac metastatic lymph node.

The question remains whether palliative resection of the primary should be proposed to patients with non-resectable metastatic adrenal cortical carcinoma, in view of potential benefit on the natural history of metastatic disease as reported for renal cell carcinoma. Indeed, a randomized controlled trial has shown that nephrectomy followed by interferon therapy resulted in longer survival among patients with metastatic renal-cell carcinoma than did interferon therapy alone (Flanigan, 2001). To our knowledge, no published report has compared the benefit of either Op'DDD therapy or palliative therapy with new anti-angiogenic monoclonal antibodies (bevacizumab) following adrenalectomy in patients with non resectable metastatic adrenal cortical carcinoma. There is furthermore limited experience and no convincing efficacy of palliative chemotherapy in advanced ACC. The best results have been achieved by the combination of etoposide, doxorubicin and cisplatin. In a recent Italian phase II trial, 10 (13%) out of 72 patients with non-resectable adrenal cortical carcinoma were amenable to radical surgery after objective response following etoposide, doxorubicin and cisplatin plus Op'DDD (Berruti, 2005).

Surgical strategy

At the time of surgery, most adrenal cortical carcinomas are large tumors with an average weight of 800 g and a mean size of 12 cm. The macroscopic appearance is usually that of a soft and hypervascular tumor, with a thin capsule and dense adhesions to adjacent organs. The principal objective of radical surgery is to achieve complete R0 resection with locoregional lymphadenectomy. All efforts should be made to avoid tumor effraction or intra-operative hemorrhage to minimize the risks of tumor seeding and locoregional recurrence. One should bear in mind the particular factors prone to tumor effraction in primary ACC: size of the tumor, anatomical location, thin capsule, dense and hypervascular adhesions to adjacent organs, fragility of tissues exposed to cortisol hypersecretion. Large surgical exposure is therefore required to ensure safe surgical resection of locally-advanced adrenal malignant tumors. In most cases, a bi-subcostal laparatomy with midline extension represents the best choice for both right and left ACC. In our experience, very large tumors may require a thoraco-abdominal approach to allow exposition and resection in a patient placed in the semi-lateral decubitus position. In that setting, abdominal incision is prolonged on the 7th or 8th rib with resection of the corresponding rib. The diaphragm should be divided peripherally rather than radially to prevent phrenic nerve injury and postoperative respiratory complications. Like others, it has been our surgical policy to perform en-bloc resection of locally-advanced ACC together with adjacent organs after primary vascular control to ensure free surgical margin, complete clearance of lumbar fossa and regional lymphadenectomy, avoid tumor effraction and minimize blood loss. Even if the tumor eventually remains microscopically confined to the adrenal gland (65% of the cases), this surgical strategy, which implies the resection of non-invaded adjacent organs is necessary for different reasons that vary according to side of the ACC: size of the tumor, constraints of exposure, tight and hypervascular adhesions to adjacent organs, left-sided portal hypertension *(figure 5)*. As a matter of fact, positive resection margins or uncontrolled hemorrhage can be expected if blunt dissection is used to separate a locally invasive tumor from periadrenal structures. True invasion to adjacent organs

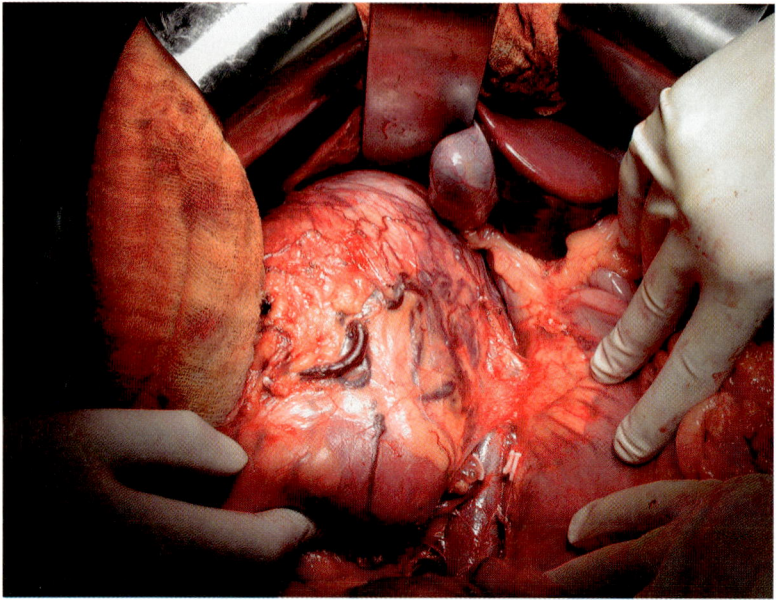

Figure 5. Stage III ACC with en-bloc resection of invaded kidney and non invaded right liver.
Figure 5a. Operative view.

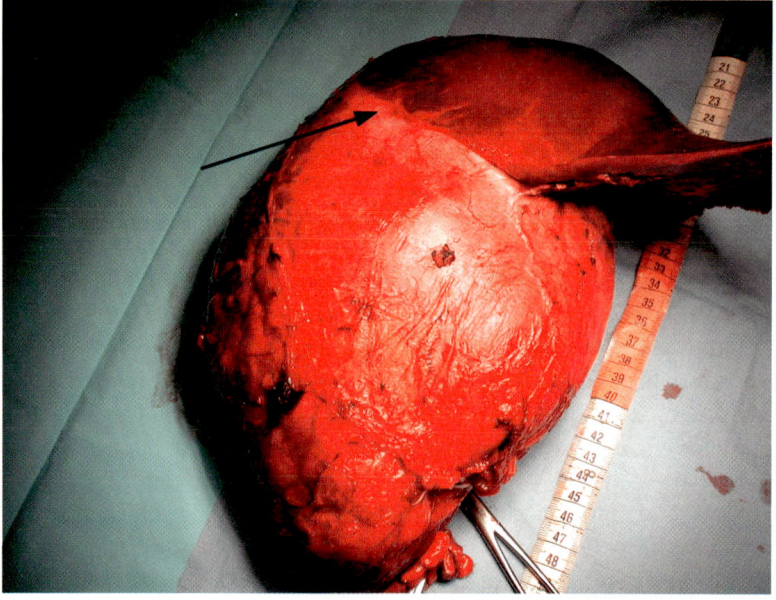

Figure 5b. Surgical specimen including right ACC, right kidney and right liver (segments V, VI, VII, VIII).
Black arrow: see dense hypervascular adhesions between ACC and right liver.

in stage III disease is therefore documented in about 35% of surgical specimen following enlarged major resections: liver, diaphragm, right colon, right kidney and duodenum for right-sided tumors; spleen, pancreas, left colon, left kidney and diaphragm for left-sided tumors *(figure 6)*. In view of extensive peri-aorto-caval dissection, a particular attention should be paid to thorough lymphostasis with liberal use of surgical clips and adequate abdominal drainage. In case of resectable liver metastases (stage IV disease), combined resection of the primary tumor and liver metastases can be selectively proposed to fit patients as the only hope for cure.

In stage III and IV disease, it has been our policy to resect the ipsilateral kidney in most cases for the aforementioned reasons, except in patients with impaired renal function or non resectable stage IV metastatic disease. In return, adrenalectomy with adjacent lymphadenectomy and upper peri-renal fat resection was the baseline surgery for stage I and small-sized (< 10 cm) stage II patients. In recent years, there has been a general agreement to preclude laparoscopic resection of primary ACC, except for incidentalomas less than 6 cm with suspicious CT and MRI findings (Saunders, 2004). Even in this setting, several reports have highlighted an increased risk of locoregional recurrence or retro- or intraperitoneal carcinomatosis (Gonzalez, 2005; Henry, 2002; Kebebew, 2002). For most endocrine surgeons, the preoperative imaging evidence of malignancy would lead to open adrenalectomy. Conversely, any intraoperative findings consistent with ACC (macroscopic appearance, dense adhesions or abnormal feeding vessels) during lapararoscopic adrenalectomy should lead to the conversion to an open procedure (Saunder, 2004). More recently, as part of an ongoing prospective study, all of our patients with an adrenal incidentaloma were submitted to a complete imaging work-up including CT scan, MRI and ^{18}FDG-PET-scan. The high diagnostic accuracy of PET scan for the diagnosis of primary ACC has led us to preclude the laparoscopic approach for any incidentaloma with increased ^{18}FDG uptake, whatever the size of the tumor (non published data).

Macroscopic venous invasion is common in primary ACC and more frequently observed in right-sided tumors with a reported incidence of 20% including right or left adrenal vein, left renal vein or inferior vena cava. Extension into the IVC represents a surgical challenge. We recently reported our experience of a 15-patient series and reviewed the literature (Chiche, 2006). Most cases of IVC invasion (85%) are represented by tumoral thrombus extension originating from a right-sided ACC (80%) without microscopic venous invasion. Direct invasion to the venous wall is often limited and can be treated by partial wedge resection and direct closure. Caval resection with graft replacement is indicated in less than 5% of the patients. In our experience, the upper level of caval extension is best documented by the combination of caval Doppler ultrasound, trans-esophageal echocardiography and angio-MRI *(figure 7)*. The upper level of caval invasion can be located below, behind or above the liver, with or without right atrial extension. Accordingly, caval thrombectomy can be performed by cross-clamping of the IVC, by hepatic vascular exclusion or by cardiopulmonary bypass with hypothermic circulatory arrest. In selected instances of caval extension above the suprahepatic veins but without atrial extension, thrombectomy can be achieved by hepatic vascular exclusion with intra-pericardic control of IVC and use of external veno-venous bypass.

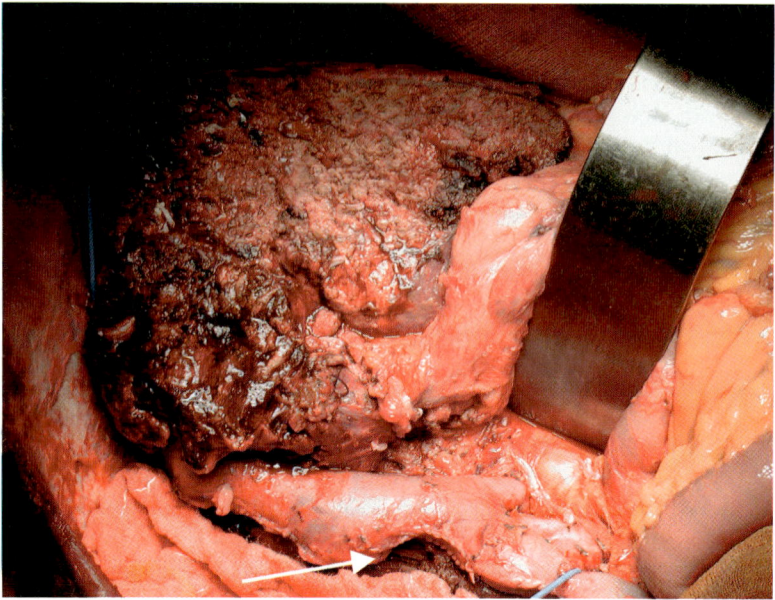

Figure 6. En-bloc resection of a stage III locally-advanced ACC together with right liver, right kidney, ileo-colon and inferior vena cava.
Figure 6a. Operative view.
White arrow. See partial vena caval resection with prosthetic polyurethane patch replacement (venous invasion + retrohepatic caval thrombus).

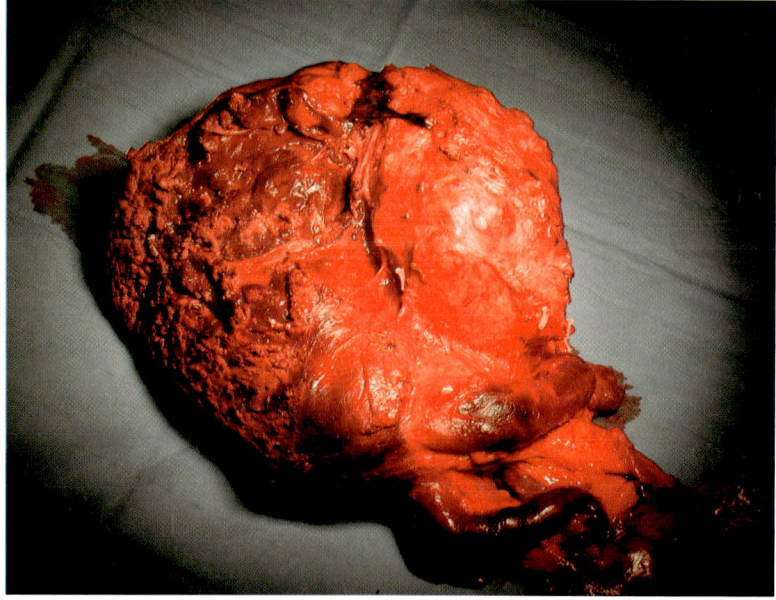

Figure 6b. Posterior view of the surgical specimen. Pathologic examination revealed contiguous extension to the liver, right colon and vena cava without positive lymph nodes or kidney involvement.

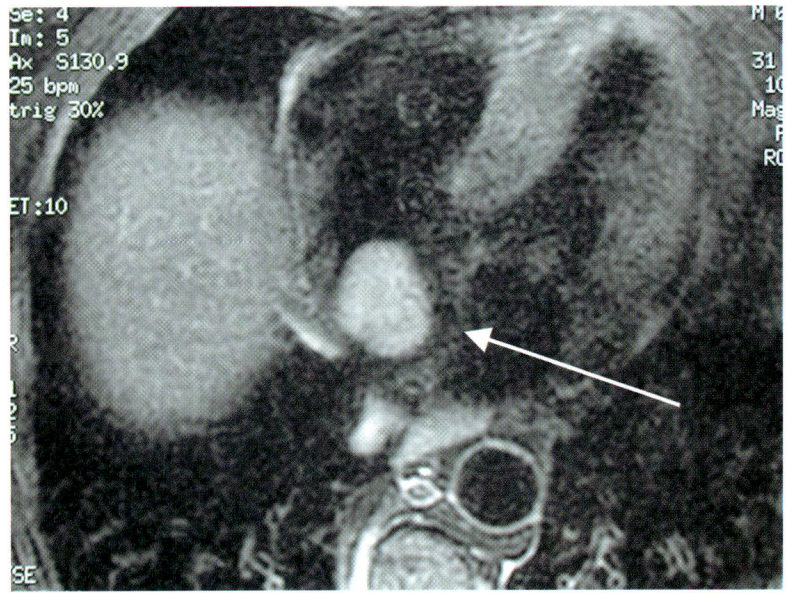

Figure 7. Right ACC with inferior vena caval invasion extending into the right atrium.
Figure 7a. *MRI showing intra-atrial extension of the tumoral thrombus into the right atrium (white arrow).*

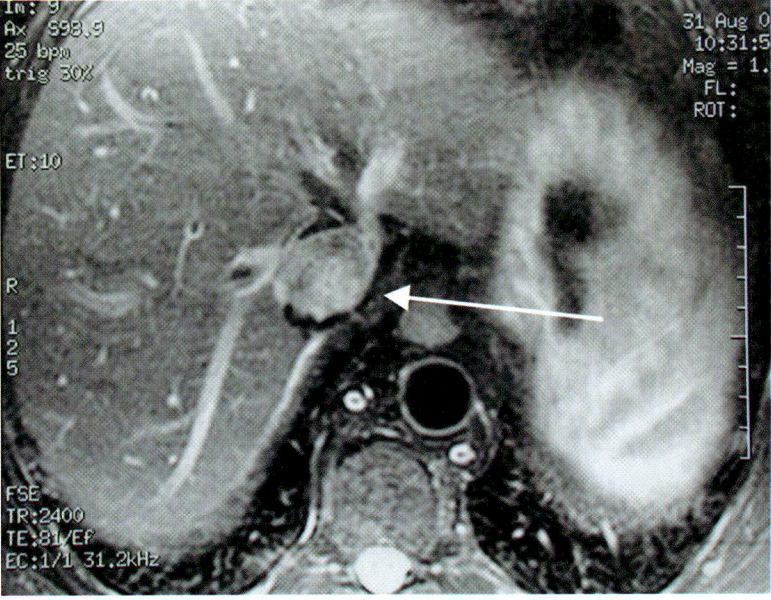

Figure 7b. *MRI showing nearly complete obstruction of the inferior vena cava above the supra-hepatic veins (same patient).*

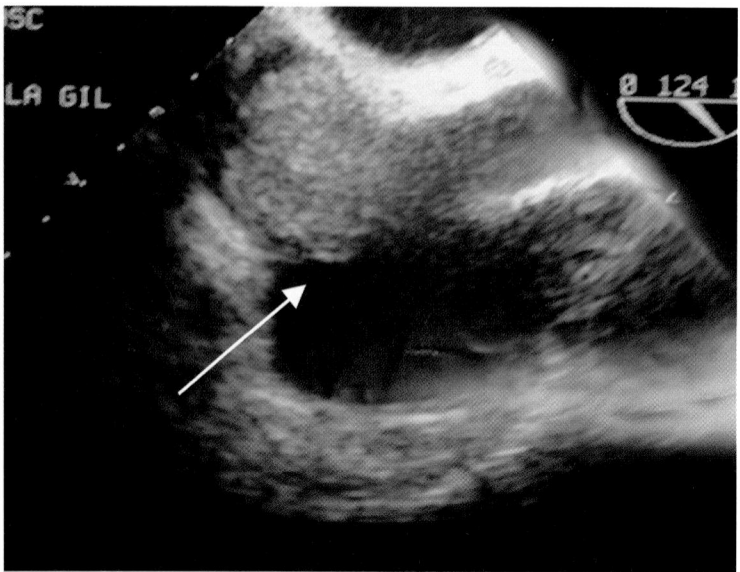

Figure 7c. *Trans-esophageal echocardiography demonstrating protruding thrombus into the right atrium (white arrow). The patient underwent thrombectomy by sterno-bi-subcostal incision under cardio-pulmonary bypass with hypothermic cardiac arrest.*

Postoperative care

It has been our practice to start a cortisol substitution intra-operatively in most patients, regardless of their secreting profile, considering that "over-substitution" was preferable to delayed diagnosis of postoperative adrenal insufficiency following major surgery. Despite careful intraoperative lymphostasis, ascitic chylous effusion is likely to occur as a result of extensive surgery together with periaortocaval dissection. Drains are therefore removed after the resumption of oral intake, and any substantial chylous leak is treated by fat-free oral regimen and prolonged abdominal drainage. Rare instances of severe ascitic chylous effusion may require parenteral nutrition together with the administration of somatostatin analogs. In metastatic stage IV ACC, there is convincing evidence that nearly 35% of patients will benefit from Op'DDD therapy provided mitotanemia is maintained above a level of 14 µg/L (Luton, 1990; Wooten, 1993; Baudin, 2001). Our group recently suggested that Op'DDD therapy is especially indicated in patients with cortisol-secreting adrenal cortical carcinoma (Abiven, 2006). We therefore propose Op'DDD therapy to all stage III and IV patients following surgery and more recently to all patients with cortisol-secreting adrenal cortical carcinoma regardless of the stage of the disease (Abiven, 2006). Most locoregional or metastatic recurrences following surgical resection of ACC arise within 2 years of surgical resection, even though late recurrences have also been described up to 14 years after surgery (Schulick, 1999; Icard, 2001). The question remains when to stop Op'DDD therapy in patients without recurrence after two years of treatment, bearing in mind the frequent side-effects of the drug, the constraints of treatment and the need for concomitant cortisol substitution.

Surgical outcome

Surgical results and long-term outcome following resection of primary ACC are summarized in *table V*. Operative mortality is ranging from 5 to 8% mostly occurring in patients with stage III or IV disease undergoing an extensive resection (Icard, 1992a; Schulick, 1999; Icard, 2001). Overall median survival is 33 months ranging from 37 to 74 months after curative resection (71-84%) and from 6 to 27 months after uncomplete surgery (16-29%) (Crucitti, 1996; Harrison, 1999; Icard, 1992a; Icard *et al.*, 2001; Vassilopoulou-Sellin, 2001, non published Cochin surgical series). The 5-year overall survival rate is 40% ranging from 34 to 46%. Besides curative resection, the principal prognostic factor is represented by the stage of the disease. The 5-year survival rate is 55-64% for stage I-II disease, 21-28% for stage III disease and 0-5% for stage IV disease (Abiven, 2006, Crucitti, 1996; Harrison, 1999; Icard, 1992a; Icard, 2001; Vassilopoulou-Sellin, 2001) Gender, size of the tumor, associated nephrectomy or lymphadenectomy had no clear impact on survival. Younger age, androgen-secreting tumors have been reported to be associated with better prognosis, whereas cortisol-secreting tumors were associated with reduced survival (Abiven, 2006; Icard, 1992a). The reported incidence of locoregional and metastatic recurrence rates ranges from 22 to 32%, and 40 to 50%, respectively.

Table V. Surgical results and long-term outcome following resection of primary adrenal cortical carcinoma according to principal series.

Centre	N cases (study period)	Stage I-II/ III-IV	Overall 5-year survival rate	Loco-regional recurrence rate	Metastatic recurrence rate	Operative mortality
MD Anderson (Vassilopoulou-Sellin, 2001)	139 (1980-2000)	33/77%	45%	–	–	–
French registry (Icard, 2001)	253 (1978-1997)	56/44%	38%	32%	50%	5.5%
Italian registry (Crucitti, 1996)	129 (1980-1995)	49/51%	35%	23%	51%	–
Mayo Clinic (Kendrick, 2001)	58 (1980-1996)	52/48%	37%	26%	40%	5%
Memorial Sloan-Kettering (Harrison, 1999)	46 (1986-1996)	–	36%	–	–	–
Cochin surgical series (personal data)	104 (1980-2002)	45/55%	46%	22%	43%	6%

Extended resection for stage III and IV disease

In the non published Cochin surgical series of 104 primary ACC, there were 30 patients with stage III disease and 27 with stage IV disease. Among these 57 patients, forty-three patients underwent ipsilateral nephrectomy and twenty patients had extended en-bloc resection of adjacent organs. In left-sided ACC (9 patients), this included 5 splenopancreatectomies, 2 splenectomies, 2 left colonic resections and 2 partial diaphragm resections. For right-sided ACC (11 patients), adjacent organ resections consisted of 3 right hepatectomies, 1 segmentectomy VI, 4 right colonic resections, 2 duodenal disk excisions, and 3 partial diaphragm resections. Curative resection was achieved in 84% of the 20 patients with extended "en bloc" resection. Two patients died from surgical complications. As stated before, microscopic invasion of adjacent resected organs was observed in 35% of the surgical specimen, and metastatic lymph nodes were present in 28% of the patients. Median survival was 26 months (6-146 months) with 13 patients surviving more than two years.

Of the 27 patients with initial metastatic disease, 13 underwent palliative resection of the primary ACC in view of non resectable multifocal metastatic spread. Fourteen patients with resectable liver metastases underwent combined hepatic and left (n = 5) or right (n = 9) ACC resection. Ipsilateral nephrectomy was associated in 13 patients. Surgery was judged complete in all instances, giving an overall curative resection rate of 52% (14/27). The hepatic resection consisted of 11 right hepatectomies, 2 left lateral lobectomies (segment II and III) and one segmentectomy VI *(figure 8)*. Two patients with vena caval extension furthermore underwent caval thrombectomy. One patient died postoperatively. Median survival was 17 months (4-56 months) with 6 patients surviving more than two years.

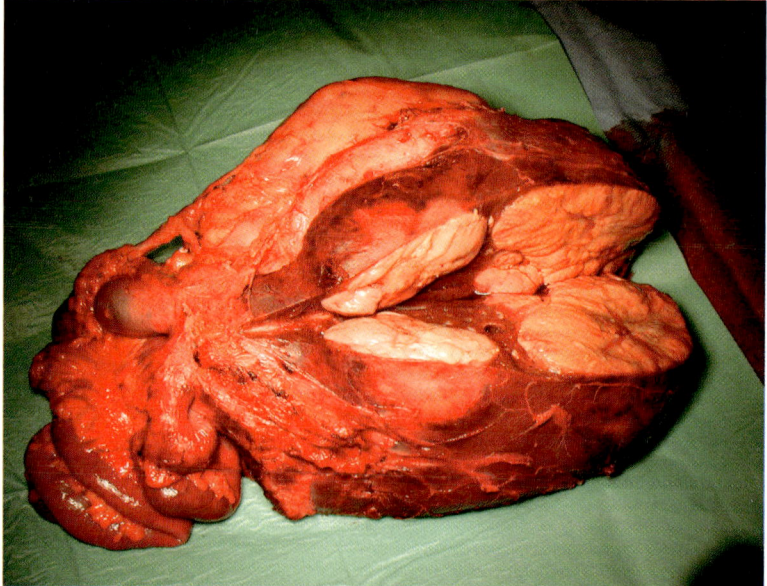

Figure 8. Right adrenal cortical carcinoma with synchronous resectable liver metastases treated by en-bloc resection of liver, kidney, ACC and ileocolon.

Surgery of recurrent adrenal cortical carcinoma and metastases

In our surgical series of 104 patients, 24 patients developed a locoregional recurrence after a median time of 17 months (6-42 months), 14 of whom were judged resectable after imaging workup. The locoregional recurrence was confined to primary surgical site (n = 9) or associated with liver metastases (n = 5) *(figure 8)*. Repeat surgery consisted of exploratory laparotomy with biopsy (n = 1), resection of local recurrence (n = 9), resection of local and liver metastatic recurrent disease (n = 4). Surgery was complete in 13/24 patients (54%), with one postoperative death and a median survival of 37 months, similar to that observed after primary resection *(figure 9)*.

40 patients developed metachronous metastases to the liver (n = 29) to the lungs (n = 26) to the bones (n = 10) or to other miscellaneous sites (n = 9 including a controlateral adrenal deposit). Metastatic recurrence was multifocal in 27 patients and occurred after a median delay of 19 months (4-76 months). Eight patients (20%) underwent complete resection of liver (n = 5), lung (n = 2) and adrenal (n = 1) metastatic disease without operative mortality. Median survival in this subgroup of patients was 29 months. Our results are similar to those of previous reports, indicating both increased survival and satisfactory survival rates in patients undergoing curative resection of recurrent ACC (Bellantone, 1997; Schulick, 1999).

Summary

Adrenal cortical carcinoma is a rare tumor with dismal prognosis. Early diagnosis and complete surgical resection is the only potential of cure. In stage I disease, all efforts should be made for accurate preoperative diagnosis, especially in patients presenting with an incidentaloma. This includes complete hormonal assessment and adequate imaging work-up including ^{18}FDG-PET scan which appears promising. In that setting, there is no place for laparoscopic surgery. Patients with stage II disease are best treated by adrenalectomy, upper peri-renal fat resection and locoregional lymphadenectomy with a 5-year survival rate of nearly 60%. In locally-advanced ACC (stage III and IV disease), the main goals of surgery are to achieve complete resection with free surgical margin and minimal blood loss, which may often requires "en-bloc" resection of non-invaded adjacent organs. In our experience, this surgical strategy both aims at increasing survival and minimizing the risks of recurrent disease. Inferior vena caval invasion furthermore represents a challenging issue, which should be managed by experienced surgical teams. Locoregional recurrence is amenable to complete surgical resection in nearly half of the cases, with a median survival time similar to that observed after primary resection whereas most metastatic recurrence will require medical palliation. It has been our policy to propose adjuvant Op'DDD therapy following resection of locally-advanced ACC, especially in patients with cortisol-secreting tumors. Further studies are needed to assess the benefits of new adjuvant therapy following surgery, such antiangiogenic monoclonal antibodies or new cytotoxic agents.

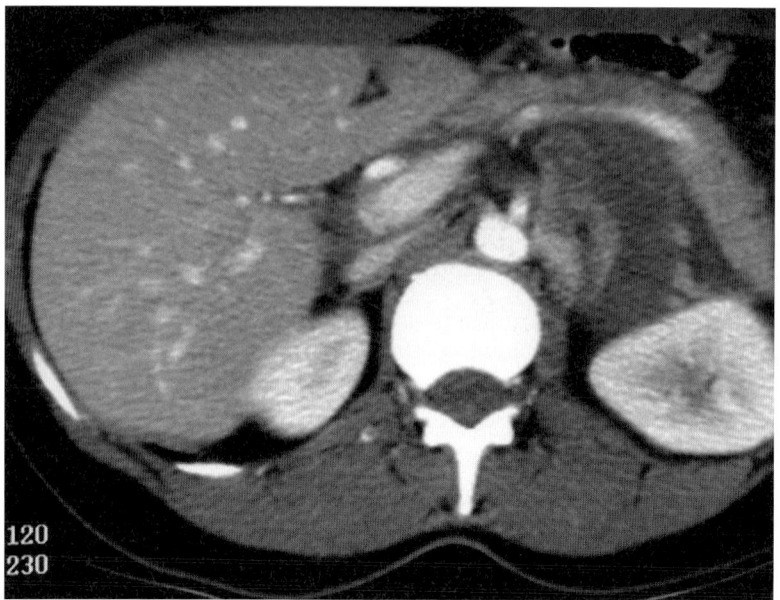

Figure 9. Locoregional recurrence following resection of left adrenal cortical carcinoma. Curative surgery included resection of local recurrence and left kidney.
Figure 9a. CT scan

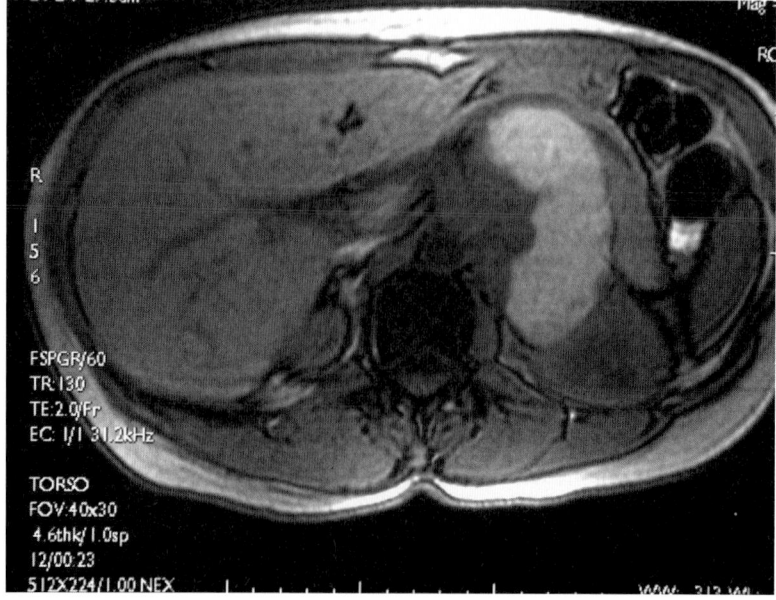

Figure 9b. MRI

References

Third National Cancer Survey: incidence Data. (1975). In *NCI monograph*, N. C. Institut (Ed.), pp. 41. Bethesda: DHEW Publ.

Abiven G, Coste J, Groussin L, et al. Clinical and biological features in the prognosis of adreno cortical carcinoma: poor outcome of cortisol-secreting tumors in a series of 202 consecutive patients. *J Clin Endocrinol Metab* 2006; 91: 2650-55.

Aubert S, Wacrenier A, Leroy X, et al. Weiss system revisited: a clinicopathologic and immunohistochemical study of 49 adrenocortical tumors. *Am J Surg Pathol* 2002; 26 (12): 1612-9.

Baudin E, Pellegriti G, Bonnay M, et al. Impact of monitoring plasma 1,1-dichlorodiphenildichloroethane (o,p'DDD) levels on the treatment of patients with adrenal cortical carcinoma. *Cancer* 2001; 92 (6): 1385-92.

Becherer A, Vierhapper H, Potzi C, et al. FDG-PET in adrenal cortical carcinoma. *Cancer Biother Radiopharm* 2001; 16 (4): 289-95.

Bellantone R, Ferrante A, Boscherini M, et al. Role of reoperation in recurrence of adrenal cortical carcinoma: results from 188 cases collected in the Italian National Registry for Adrenal Cortical Carcinoma. *Surgery* 1997; 122 (6): 1212-8.

Berruti A, Terzolo M, Sperone P, et al. Etoposide, doxorubicin and cisplatin plus Op'DDD in the treatment of advanced adrenal cortical carcinoma: a large prospective phase II trial. *Endocr Relat Cancer* 2005; 12 (3): 657-66.

Boland GW, Lee MJ, Gazelle GS, Halpern EF, McNicholas MM, Mueller PR. Characterization of adrenal masses using unenhanced CT: an analysis of the CT literature. *AJR Am J Roentgenol* 1998; 171 (1): 201-4.

Chiche L, Dousset B, Kieffer E, Chapuis Y. Adrenal cortical carcinoma extending into the inferior vena cava: Presentation of a 15-patient series and review of the literature. *Surgery* 2006; 139 (1): 15-27.

Crucitti F, Bellantone R, Ferrante A, Boscherini M, Crucitti P. The Italian Registry for Adrenal Cortical Carcinoma: analysis of a multiinstitutional series of 129 patients. The ACC Italian Registry Study Group. *Surgery* 1996; 119 (2): 161-70.

Dackiw AP, Lee JE, Gagel RF, Evans DB. Adrenal cortical carcinoma. *World J Surg* 2001; 25 (7): 914-26.

Flanigan RC, Salmon SE, Blumenstein BA, et al. Nephrectomy followed by interferon alfa-2b compared with interferon alfa-2b alone for metastatic renal-cell cancer. *N Engl J Med* 2001; 345 (23): 1655-9.

Gicquel C, Bertagna X, Schneid H, et al. Rearrangements at the 11p15 locus and overexpression of insulin-like growth factor-II gene in sporadic adrenocortical tumors. *J Clin Endocrinol Metab* 1994a; 78 (6): 1444-53.

Gicquel C, Bertherat J, Le Bouc Y, Bertagna X. Pathogenesis of adrenocortical incidentalomas and genetic syndromes associated with adrenocortical neoplasms. *Endocrinol Metab Clin North Am* 2000; 29 (1): 1-13, vii.

Gicquel C, Le Bouc Y. Molecular markers for malignancy in adrenocortical tumors. *Horm Res* 1997; 47 (4-6): 269-72.

Gicquel C, Leblond-Francillard M, Bertagna X, et al. Clonal analysis of human adrenal cortical carcinomas and secreting adenomas. *Clin Endocrinol (Oxf)* 1994b; 40 (4): 465-77.

Gonzalez RJ, Shapiro S, Sarlis N, et al. Laparoscopic resection of adrenal cortical carcinoma: a cautionary note. *Surgery* 2005; 138 (6): 1078-85; discussion 1085-6.

Harrison LE, Gaudin PB, Brennan MF. Pathologic features of prognostic significance for adrenal cortical carcinoma after curative resection. *Arch Surg* 1999; 134 (2): 181-5.

Henry JF, Sebag F, Iacobone M, Mirallie E. Results of laparoscopic adrenalectomy for large and potentially malignant tumors. *World J Surg* 2002; 26 (8): 1043-7.

Honigschnabl S, Gallo S, Niederle B, et al. How accurate is MR imaging in characterisation of adrenal masses: update of a long-term study. *Eur J Radiol* 2002; 41 (2): 113-22.

Icard P, Chapuis Y, Andreassian B, Bernard A, Proye C. Adrenal cortical carcinoma in surgically treated patients: a retrospective study on 156 cases by the French Association of Endocrine Surgery. *Surgery* 1992a; 112 (6): 972-9; discussion 979-80.

Icard P, Goudet P, Charpenay C, et al. Adrenal cortical carcinomas: surgical trends and results of a 253-patient series from the French Association of Endocrine Surgeons study group. *World J Surg* 2001; 25 (7): 891-7.

Icard P, Louvel A, Chapuis Y. Survival rates and prognostic factors in adrenal cortical carcinoma. *World J Surg* 1992b; 16 (4): 753-8.

Kebebew E, Siperstein AE, Clark OH, Duh QY. Results of laparoscopic adrenalectomy for suspected and unsuspected malignant adrenal neoplasms. *Arch Surg* 2002; 137 (8): 948-51; discussion 952-3.

King DR, Lack EE. Adrenal cortical carcinoma: a clinical and pathologic study of 49 cases. *Cancer* 1979; 44 (1): 239-44.

Korobkin M, Brodeur FJ, Francis IR, Quint LE, Dunnick NR, Londy F. CT time-attenuation washout curves of adrenal adenomas and nonadenomas. *AJR Am J Roentgenol* 1998; 170 (3): 747-52.

Korobkin M, Giordano TJ, Brodeur FJ, et al. Adrenal adenomas: relationship between histologic lipid and CT and MR findings. *Radiology* 1996; 200 (3): 743-7.

Luton JP, Cerdas S, Billaud L, et al. Clinical features of adrenal cortical carcinoma, prognostic factors, and the effect of Op'DDD therapy. *N Engl J Med* 1990; 322 (17): 1195-201.

Outwater EK, Siegelman ES, Huang AB, Birnbaum BA. Adrenal masses: correlation between CT attenuation value and chemical shift ratio at MR imaging with in-phase and opposed-phase sequences. *Radiology* 1996; 200 (3): 749-52.

Pommier RF, Brennan MF. An eleven-year experience with adrenal cortical carcinoma. *Surgery* 1992; 112 (6): 963-70; discussion 970-1.

Prager G, Heinz-Peer G, Passler C, et al. Can dynamic gadolinium-enhanced magnetic resonance imaging with chemical shift studies predict the status of adrenal masses? *World J Surg* 2002; 26 (8): 958-64.

Ross NS, Aron DC. Hormonal evaluation of the patient with an incidentally discovered adrenal mass. *N Engl J Med* 1990; 323 (20): 1401-5.

Saunders BD, Doherty GM. Laparoscopic adrenalectomy for malignant disease. *Lancet Oncol* 2004; 5 (12): 718-26.

Schulick RD, Brennan MF. Long-term survival after complete resection and repeat resection in patients with adrenal cortical carcinoma. *Ann Surg Oncol* 1999; 6 (8): 719-26.

Sullivan M, Boileau M, Hodges CV. Adrenal cortical carcinoma. *J Urol* 1978; 120 (6): 660-5.

Tenenbaum F, Groussin L, Foehrenbach H, et al. 18F-fluorodeoxyglucose positron emission tomography as a diagnostic tool for malignancy of adrenocortical tumours? Preliminary results in 13 consecutive patients. *Eur J Endocrinol* 2004; 150 (6): 789-92.

Terzolo M, Ali A, Osella G, Mazza E. Prevalence of adrenal carcinoma among incidentally discovered adrenal masses. A retrospective study from 1989 to 1994. Gruppo Piemontese Incidentalomi Surrenalici. *Arch Surg* 1997; 132 (8): 914-9.

Vassilopoulou-Sellin R, Schultz PN. Adrenal cortical carcinoma. Clinical outcome at the end of the 20th century. *Cancer* 2001; 92 (5): 1113-21.

Venkatesh S, Hickey RC, Sellin RV, Fernandez JF, Samaan NA. Adrenal cortical carcinoma. *Cancer* 1989; 64 (3): 765-9.

Wajchenberg BL, Albergaria Pereira MA, Medonca BB, *et al*. Adrenal cortical carcinoma: clinical and laboratory observations. *Cancer* 2000; 88 (4): 711-36.

Weiss LM. Comparative histologic study of 43 metastasizing and nonmetastasizing adrenocortical tumors. *Am J Surg Pathol* 1984; 8 (3): 163-9.

Wooten MD, King DK. Adrenal cortical carcinoma. Epidemiology and treatment with Op'DDD and a review of the literature. *Cancer* 1993; 72 (11): 3145-55.

Local treatment of adrenal cortical carcinoma metastases with interventional radiology techniques

Thiery de Baere
Radiology Department, Gustave Roussy Institute, Villejuif

Due to the low efficacy of general treatment of adrenal cortical carcinoma (ACC) and its metastases, there is frequent indication for loco-regional treatment. Loco-regional treatments have been used for many years in cancer management, including radiation therapy, brachytherapy, regional chemotherapy delivery (intra-arterial, intra-peritoneal), and obviously surgery. These treatments can provide dramatic results and cure the patient on some occasions when the disease is limited. However, the drawback of any local or regional treatment is the occurrence of new metastases in the same organ or in a distant organ. Loco-regional treatment can be provided by image guided therapy. In this setting, imaging is used to get closer to the tumor(s) and deliver the treatment to them, aiming at local or regional control of cancer.

Treatment can target a tumor directly through a direct percutaneous access for radiofrequency ablation (RFA), or can target an organ through intra-arterial drug delivery, namely trans-arterial chemoembolization of liver metastases, both described in this chapter.

Radiofrequency ablation (RFA)

RFA has achieved impressive results in the treatment of unresectable primary liver cancer (Livraghi, 1999) and liver metastases (Solbiati, 2001; de Baere, 2000). Even if the literature deals mostly with hepatocellular carcinomas and liver metastases from colorectal cancer, there are a few series dealing with less common liver metastases such as neuroendocrine tumors (Berber, 2002), and no differences in local efficacy of RFA have been demonstrated in various types of metastases. RFA has been used more recently to treat cancers at other sites, namely lungs, where several experimental studies have demonstrated that RFA can completely destroy lesions in animal tumor models (Miao, 2001). Some small and medium size clinical series have also been performed on lung, demonstrating complete tumor destruction (de Baere, 2006). Additionally, radiofrequency is used for palliative treatment of painful bone metastases (Goetz, 2004), and small series of ACCs have been reported.

Principle and technique

The goal of radiofrequency is to destroy tumors by heating cells over 60 °C in order to obtain non reversible cellular modifications. Radiofrequency (RF) is a sinusoidal current with a frequency of 400 to 500 KHz that heats tissues through ionic agitation (McGahan, 1990). To increase the RF-ablated volume by one RF delivery, the single-needle electrode has been transformed into more complex tools: expandable multiprong, cooled needles. The expandable needle is a needle containing 8 to 12 electrodes that are extended in the targeted tissue once punctured *(figure 1)*. These electrodes produce as many small areas of destruction as the number of electrodes and a larger area of destruction is achieved by combining the small areas.

Technique for ablating tumors is similar to that used for biopsies, though the procedure involves a larger caliber needle: around 14 Gauge. The RF needle-electrode is inserted under image guidance, taking advantage of the imaging to better visualize the targeted tumor. Most often, ultrasound will be used for liver tumor due to its real time ability, its availability, and multiple angulation possibilities. When a liver tumor is not seen under ultrasound, CT can be used. For lung and bone tumors RFA, CT guidance will be mandatory to guide needle insertion because it is the

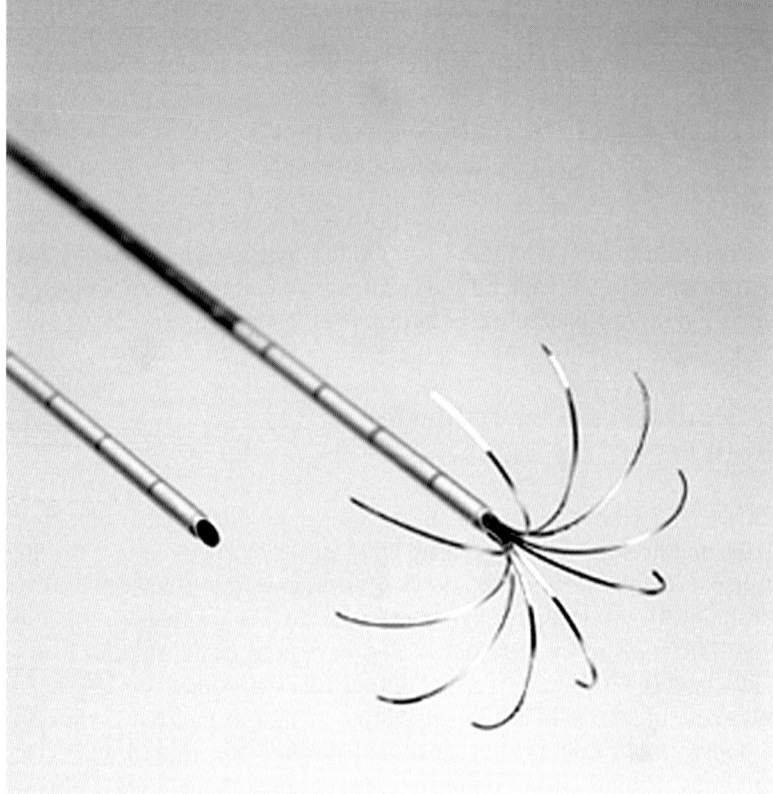

Figure 1. Distal tip of a radiofrequency needle-electrode, before expansion of the tine-electrodes (left), and after expansion of the 10 electrodes (right).

only imaging technique able to accurately see and locate at the same time tumor and needle position. The needle tract should be as short as possible and the number of needle paths should be limited as well to decrease bleeding and the likelihood of pneumothorax in lung RFA.

Patients must have normal coagulation parameters and platelet count. Several tumors can be treated during the same session, and ablation of liver and lung metastases can be performed during the same session. However, lungs should be treated one at a time to avoid the possibility of life-threatening complications from bilateral adverse events, such as massive hemorrhage or pneumothorax.

Treatment can be performed under conscious sedation or general anasthesia, but we prefer general anesthesia which allows complete immobilization of the patient and consequently will probably increase accuracy of RF needle placement in the target tumor and, as a result, increase efficacy.

Assessing the efficacy of RFA

Magnetic Resonance Imaging (MRI) and CT are the most commonly used imaging techniques (Dromain, 2002). The RF-induced lesion or "scar" should ideally be larger than the treated tumor, thus encompassing the tumor and safety margins. This scar will decrease in size albeit very slowly. Evidence of treatment efficacy is sought on early follow-up imaging.

On CT, a hypoattenuating or hyperattenuating, well delimited, round or oval scar is depicted, that is not enhanced after injection of contrast medium. On MRI T2-weighted images, scar appears homogenous and most often hypointense; on T1-weighted images, it is hypo- or hyperintense, and sometimes heterogeneous, but never exhibits enhancement after injection of gadolinium. Residual foci of active tumor are usually found at the periphery of the RF-induced lesion, more rarely an overall increase in size will reveal incomplete treatment. Foci of active tumor are usually hypo- or hyperattenuating on CT, hypointense on T1-weighted MRI, moderately hyperintense on T2-weighted images, usually demonstrating contrast enhancement. Before one to three months, it is sometimes an arduous task to differentiate contrast enhancement due to inflammatory reaction from residual tumor, thus the first imaging studies are usually performed one to three months after RFA.

In lung, CT obtained within a few minutes after the end of RF delivery shows the lung tumor surrounded by ground glass opacity, thus enlarging the diameter of the hyperattenuating area *(figure 2)*. This enlargement is even greater at 24/48 hours with lung opacity doubling in diameter. This opacity will become even more hyperattenuating and will decrease in size during follow-up.

CT imaging after ablation of bone tumors depicts very late changes; but early pain relief, which usually occurs in less than a week, is the best evidence that therapy has been successful.

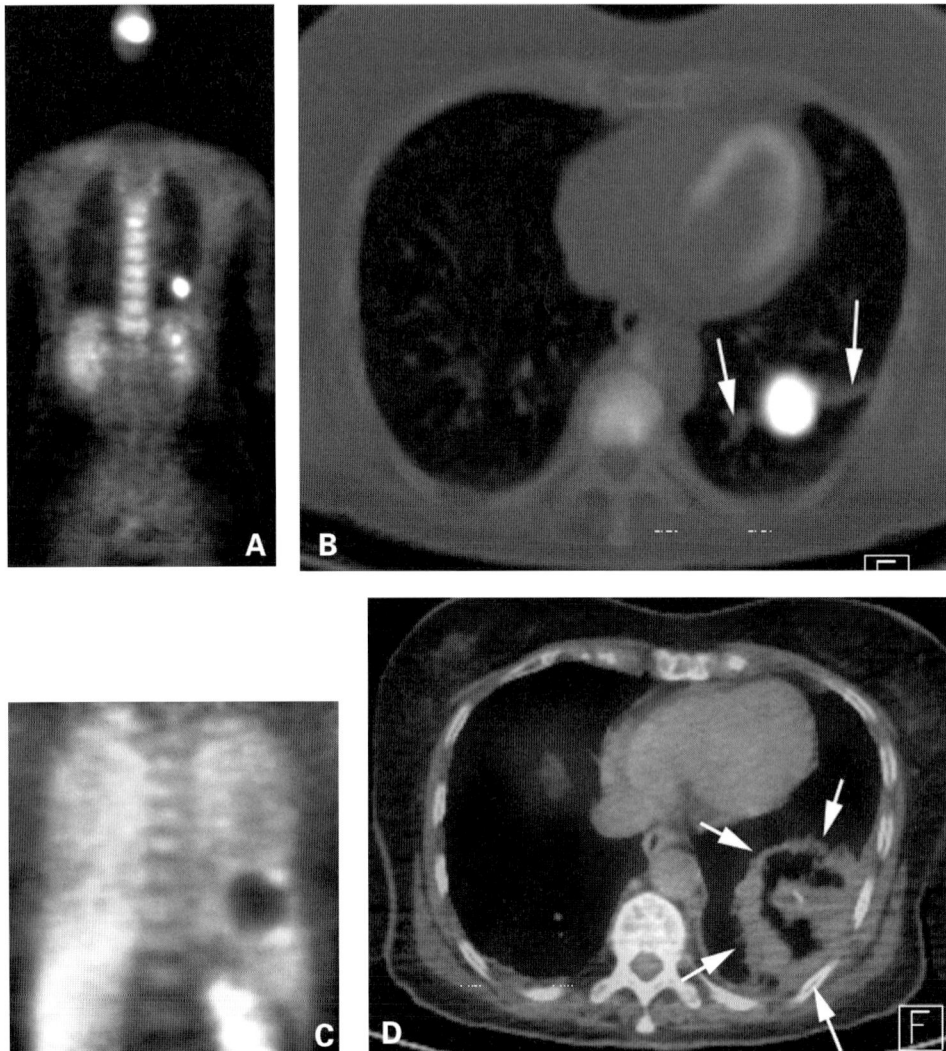

Figure 2. 2A Frontal view of a PET imaging demonstrated uptake in the lower lobe of the left lung.
2B On this fusion imaging (CT + PET) obtained in the axial plane, the uptake is demonstrated to be due to a lung metastasis from adrenal carcinoma. One can notice that the metastasis is a recurrence occurring on the scar of a previous surgery (arrows).
2C Frontal view of a PET imaging obtained one day after radiofrequency ablation of the left lower lobe metastasis demonstrating no more abnormal glucose uptake.
2D On this fusion imaging (CT + PET) obtained in the axial plane one day after radiofrequency ablation of the left lower lobe metastasis, there is no more glucose uptake. The CT image shows the opacity around the initial location of the metastasis (arrows) corresponding to the external boarder of the ablated tissue.

Indications

RF treatment can be used for ACC metastases to the liver or the lung. However, RFA should probably be limited to patients in whom surgery is contraindicated. Today, there is no large randomized trial demonstrating that RFA is as efficient as surgery, particularly in terms of patient survival. However, we demonstrated in a restrospective study of RFA in colorectal carcinoma liver metastases occurring in a patient who had already had a first hepatectomy, that survival after RFA or a second hepatectomy produced no differences in survival (Elias, 2002). Moreover, local efficacy of RFA in colorectal liver metastases were shown to be equivalent to wedge resection (Elias, 2004).

Results

There is no specific series dealing with liver metastases from ACCs treated with RFA, but no difference in RFA efficacy has been demonstrated according to tumor histology when treating liver metastases. For liver tumor including mainly hepatocellular carcinoma and metastasis, the local efficacy of RFA ranged from 60.9 to 96.4%. Reported results are very heterogeneous, probably due to differences in tumor selection, assessment criteria for efficacy and the duration of follow-up in the different series.

Whatever the series, tumor size is a major predictive factor of efficacy. Coagulation necrosis is usually achieved in more than 90% of tumors measuring less than 25 mm (Livraghi, 1999; de Baere, 2000; Song, 2001). In contrast, only 71% of tumors measuring 3 to 5 cm in diameter, and 25% of tumors 5 to 9 cm in diameter are cured with RFA (Livraghi, 2000). Consequently, tumors measuring less than 3.5 cm in diameter are the best indications for RF treatment.

For lung metastases RFA, due to the novelty of the technique, the number of patients treated is lower, but results seem close to those reported for the liver. Specific reports about RFA of ACC metastases to the lung do not exist, but in our experience with various types of metastases, including two patients with ACC metastases, we have observed treatment efficacy in 92 of 98 tumors with a minimal follow-up of 18 months (de Baere, 2006). However, local tumor recurrences were reported more than six months after treatment. These late discoveries of recurrence emphasize the interest of a preliminary report suggesting that PET scanning could be used for follow-up, allowing early detection of incomplete treatment (Antoch, 2005) *(figure 2)*.

In our series (de Baere, 2006), pneumothorax occurred in 50% of treatment sessions, but 29% were small enough not to require any treatment. The remaining 21% were expelled manually after inserting a small bore needle catheter with side-holes while the patient was still lying on the CT table, immediately after or during RFA. Finally, chest tube drainage was necessary in 9% of RFA sessions.

RFA of adrenocortical carcinoma has been reported in small series. Wood (2003) treated 15 tumors including: 5 local recurrences to the adrenal bed, 2 local recurrences invading the kidney and 2 paraspinal local recurrences, 5 liver metastases and 1 bone metastasis. They reported success in 11 of 15 tumors (Wood, 2003). Reasonable success rates have recently been reported at international conferences for treatment of adrenal tumors, in small groups of patients: eleven of thirteen various adrenal neoplasms, including eleven metastases, one pheochromocytoma and one aldosteronoma, have been RF ablated successfully (Mayo-Smith, 2004). Moreover, recently uncontrolled hypertension and hypokalemia linked to primary hyperaldosteronism with left adrenal adenoma has been reported to be successfully treated with RFA (Al-Shaikh, 2004).

RFA is used also in bone metastases for palliation of pain caused by large tumors refractory to medication and radiation therapy (Goetz, 2004). In this setting, RFA demonstrated very good results, in a multicenter trial with 43 patients presenting 1.4 to 18 cm bone metastases that were the cause of a severe pain: score of 7.9 on a scale ranging from 1 to 10, with pain refractory to radiation therapy in 74% of cases. The patients experienced pain relief representing 3 points in 40% of cases after one week, in 55% of cases after 3 weeks, and in 84% of cases at some time during follow-up. When RFA is used to manage pain, the goal is to destroy nerve endings in the endosteum, which are at least partially responsible for pain through stimulation activated by chemical agents (e.g. prostaglandins, bradykinin, substance P or histamine) released from the destroyed bone. On the other hand, because nerves are very heat sensitive, and especially the spinal cord, extreme caution should be exercised when treating the vertebral body. When posterior wall cortical bone is not present in a vertebral body tumor that is less than 1 cm from the spine, RFA may not be an option.

Transarterial chemoembolization (TACE) of liver metastases

Principle

Intra-arterial injection takes advantage of liver vascularization being 30% arterial and 70% portal, while tumors growing in the liver are nearly exclusively fed by arterial blood. Thus, a drug injected into the hepatic artery will preferentially reach the tumor.

In fact, during TACE, chemotherapy is emulsified with Lipiodol®, because oil drops injected in the arterial flow have a propensity to go through the largest arteries without entering the small ones (de Baere, 1995). Because hypervascular tumors have larger vessels lipiodol will go preferentially to the tumors. This selectivity to the tumor is measured in an experimental model to be between 4 and 10 fold higher than for normal liver (de Baere, 1996). Embolization after chemo-lipiodol increases the efficacy of treatment by providing additional ischemia to the highly hypervascularized tumor usually targeted with this treatment. Such embolization has been reported to induce failure of transmenbrane pump, thus increasing drug retention inside the cells (Kruskal, 1993).

Indications

TACE can be performed when disease is only located in the liver or predominant in the liver, and consequently life expectancy is related to liver metastases control.

In metastatic disease, liver is often a stepwise pattern of metastatic progression and local treatment will often be associated with systemic treatment to prevent spread of disease to other organs. TACE is indicated for secondary liver tumors when they are not surgical candidates. TACE is considered as a palliative treatment even if some cases of complete and prolonged responses to treatment have been observed. TACE ranks second behind RFA which is considered a curative treatment. Consequently, TACE is proposed to patient not amenable to surgery or radiofrequency.

TACE has been reported to provide high response rate in tumors with predominant arterial feeding such as hepatocellular carcinoma and metastases from neuroendocrine tumors (Roche, 2003). On the other hand, colorectal cancer metastases demonstrated a poor arterial supply and poor response to TACE. Consequently, best candidates are hypervascular tumors.

The size and the number of tumors are of importance. Indeed, for primary liver tumor and for neuroendocrine tumors, where TACE has been used extensively, it appears that better response and less toxicity are obtained in patient with lower tumor burden. Less than 30% of tumor involvement of the liver is preferable (Roche, 2003). When tumor load is important, usually two successive courses of TACE, performed successively in the right and left part of the liver, are performed six to eight weeks apart to avoid major side effects, namely liver function alteration. Propylaxis with antibiotic (clavulanate 2g per day) started the day of the TACE and prolonged for four days is usual to prevent potential infection. TACE is contra-indicated in patient presenting a bilioenteric anastomosis or dilation of bile ducts, due to high risk of sepsis, with liver abscess formation due to bile duct contamination (de Baere, 1996). Liver insufficiency is obviously a contra-indication, and a tumor involvement of more than 60% when treating metastases from neuroendocrine tumor increases the risk of complication (Roche, 2003). Portal vein must patent to allow for arterial embolization.

Assessing the efficacy of TACE *(figure 3)*

There is no specific report of TACE for liver metastases of ACCs in the literature.

We have treated 20 patients without major complications and we have the follow-up for 12 patients with progressive metastatic liver disease proven by increase in size of liver metastases on two subsequent CT imagings. Eight of these patients were progressive after one line (n = 4) or two lines (n = 4) of chemotherapy. After one to four sessions of TACE per patient, partial response was achieved in three patients (25%), disease stabilization was possible in five patients (42%) and progression was seen in four patients (33%). Mean duration of response or stabilization was 5.3 months (range: 1-10 months). On a tumor by tumor basis, out of 44 tumors, we obtained nine complete responses, five partial responses and 19 stabilizations. It is noteworthy that

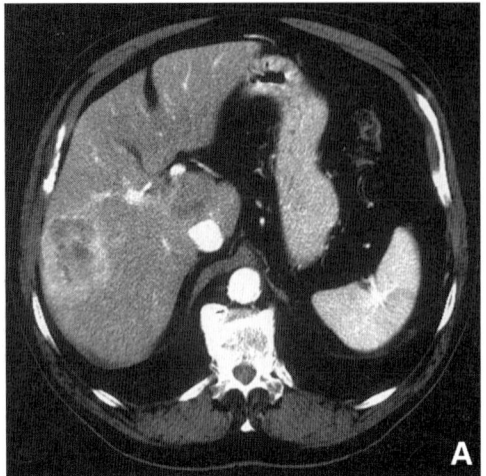
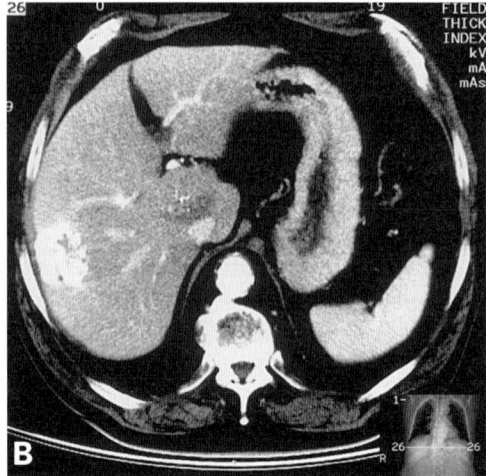
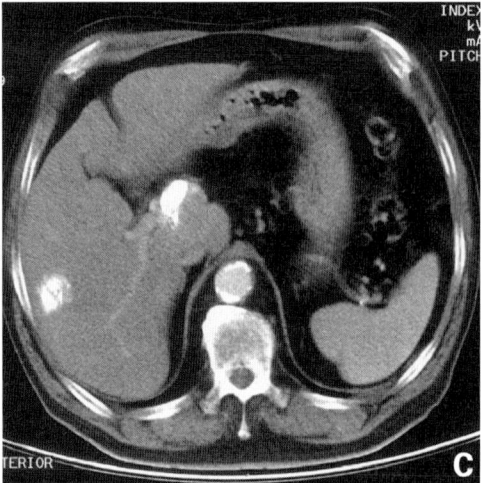

Figure 3. 3A CT scan obtained at the arterial phase demonstrates a hypervascular metastasis from ACC in the right lobe of the liver and a second metastasis of segment I.
3B: CT scan obtained with contrast injection two months after one course of TACE shows Lipiodol uptake in a tumor which slightly decreased in size of the right liver tumor.
3B: CT scan obtained without contrast injection six months after one course of TACE shows Lipiodol uptake in right liver and segment I tumors which demonstrated partial response to treatment.

complete response always occurred in metastases smaller than 3 cm, and consequently TACE had to be proposed as early as possible. A decrease of more than 50% in hormone level was noted in three out of eight evaluated patients with secreting tumors.

After TACE, there is always an increase in transaminases from two fold normal value up to ten times. Fever (grade 2-3), nausea or vomiting (grade 2-3), and a certain degree of malaise were found in 65% of TACE-treated patients, and are considered a usual post-embolization syndrome.

Conclusion

Local treatment by image guided therapy can provide control of adrenal tumors and liver or lung metastases. Most often, these treatments are effective in patients with low tumor burden and consequently must be proposed early during the disease. Due to the small size of the series, there is no proof of survival benefit, and further investigations are needed.

References

Al-Shaikh AA, Al-Rawas MM, Al-Asnag MA. Primary hyperaldosteronism treated by radiofrequency ablation. *Saudi Med J* 2004; 25: 1711-4.

Antoch G, Vogt FM, Veit, P, *et al*. Assessment of liver tissue after radiofrequency ablation: findings with different imaging procedures. *J Nucl Med* 2005; 46: 520-5.

Berber E, Flesher N, Siperstein AE. Laparoscopic radiofrequency ablation of neuroendocrine liver metastases. *World J Surg* 2002; 26: 985-90.

de Baere T, Dufaux J, Roche A, *et al*. Circulatory alterations induced by intra-arterial injection of iodized oil and emulsions of iodized oil and Doxorubicin: Experimental study. *Radiology* 1995; 194: 165-70.

de Baere T, Roche A, Amenabar JM, *et al*. Liver abscess formation after local treatment of liver tumors. *Hepatology* 1996; 23: 1436-40.

de Baere T, Zhang X, Aubert B, *et al*. Quantification of tumor uptake of iodized oils and emulsions of iodized oils: Experimental study. *Radiology* 1996; 731-5.

de Baere T, Elias D, Dromain C, *et al*. Radiofrequency ablation of 100 hepatic metastases with a mean follow-up of more than 1 year. *AJR* 2000; 175: 1619-25.

de Baere T, Palussiere J, Auperin A, *et al*. Prospective evaluation of mid-term local efficacy and survival after radio-frequency ablation of lung tumors with a minimum follow-up of 1 year. *Radiology* 2006; in press.

Dromain C, de Baere T, Elias D, *et al*. Hepatic tumors treated with percutaneous radiofrequency ablation: CT and MR Imaging Follow-up. *Radiology* 2002; 223: 255-62.

Elias D, De Baere T, Smayra T, Ouellet JF, Roche A, Lasser P. Percutaneous radiofrequency thermoablation as an alternative to surgery for treatment of liver tumor recurrence after hepatectomy. *Br J Surg* 2002; 89: 752-6.

Elias D, Baton O, Sideris L, Matsuhisa T, Pocard M, Lasser P. Local recurrences after intraoperative radiofrequency ablation of liver metastases: a comparative study with anatomic and wedge resections. *Ann Surg Oncol* 2004; 11: 500-5.

Goetz MP, Callstrom MR, Charboneau JW, *et al*. Percutaneous image-guided radiofrequency ablation of painful metastases involving bone: a multicenter study. *J Clin Oncol* 2004; 22: 300-6.

Kruskal JB, Hlatky L, Hahnfeldt P, Teramoto K, Stokes KR, Clouse ME. In vivo and *in vitro* analysis of the effectiveness of doxorubicin combined with temporary arterial occlusion in liver tumors. *J Vasc Interv Radiol* 1993; 4: 741-7.

Livraghi T, Goldberg S, Lazzaroni S, Meloni F, Solbiaiti L, Gazelle S. Small hepatocellular carcinoma: treatment with radiofrequency ablation versus ethanol injection. *Radiology* 1999; 210: 655-61.

Livraghi T, Goldberg SN, Lazzaroni S, *et al*. Hepatocellular carcinoma: radio-frequency ablation of medium and large lesions. *Radiology* 2000; 214: 761-8.

Mayo-Smith WW, Dupuy DE. Adrenal neoplasms: CT-guided radiofrequency ablation – preliminary results. *Radiology* 2004; 231: 225-30.

McGahan J, Browning P, Brock J, Teslik H. Hepatic ablation using radiofrequency electrocautery. *Invest Radiol* 1990; 25: 267-70.

Miao Y, Ni Y, Bosmans H, *et al*. Radiofrequency ablation for eradication of pulmonary tumor in rabbits. *J Surg Res* 2001; 99: 265-71.

Roche A, Girish BV, de Baere T, *et al*. Trans-catheter arterial chemoembolization as first-line treatment for hepatic metastases from endocrine tumors. *Eur Radiol* 2003; 13: 136-40.

Solbiati L, Livraghi T, Goldberg SN, *et al*. Percutaneous radio-frequency ablation of hepatic metastases from colorectal cancer: long-term results in 117 patients. *Radiology* 2001; 221: 159-66.

Song SY, Chung JW, Han JK, *et al*. Liver abscess after transcatheter oily chemoembolization for hepatic tumors: incidence, predisposing factors, and clinical outcome. *J Vasc Interv Radiol* 2001; 12: 313-20.

Wood BJ, Abraham J, Hvizda JL, Alexander HR, Fojo T. Radiofrequency ablation of adrenal tumors and adrenocortical carcinoma metastases. *Cancer* 2003; 97: 554-60.

Scintigraphic Explorations in Adrenal Cortical Carcinomas

Florence Tenenbaum
Nuclear Medicine Department, Cochin Hospital, Paris

For the investigation of adrenocortical tumors, two major questions can be approached by nuclear medicine:

1 – Could a hypersecretory or non-hypersecretory adrenal mass be an adrenal cortical carcinoma (ACC)?

2 – When an ACC is diagnosed, how to evaluate its extension, and eventually perform a whole body scan in nuclear medicine?

The first adrenotropic radiopharmaceuticals for scintigraphic explorations have been in use since the end of the 1960's. Two radiopharmaceuticals are currently available:

– A cholesterol analogue labelled with iodine 131, specific to the adrenal cortex.

– ^{18}F-fluorodeoxyglucose (FDG), a non-specific PET tracer, which is used in a wide variety of malignant tumors.

– For the future, new PET tracers are under evaluation, among them, ^{11}C-metomidate, specific to the adrenal cortex.

Adrenocortical Scintigraphy with Iodocholesterol

Cholesterol is a precursor to steroid biosynthesis and its concentration is highest in the adrenal cortex. Thus, when labelled with a gamma emitter it can be used as a radiopharmaceutical. Several molecules have been synthesised among which ^{131}I-6-iodomethyl-19-norcholesterol (NP59), a cholesterol analogue, has shown the highest concentrations in the adrenal cortex, without increasing background activity (Beierwalters, 1978; Sarkar, 1977).

Principle

This is a diagnostic imaging procedure. The radiopharmaceutical used in France and the United States is NP 59. In other European countries, a similar analogue labelled with Selenium

75 is used. Results from these two tracers are comparable (Shapiro, 1981). NP 59 is a cholesterol analogue which is integrated into low density lipoproteins (LDL). Via LDL receptors, a small percentage enters the cells of the three zones (glomerulosa, fasciculata and reticularis) of the adrenal cortex. Uptake is stimulated by ACTH and angiotensin II. It is then stored in the cells in its esterified form. After its incorporation into LDLs, the radiopharmaceutical is primarily metabolized by the liver, especially by biliary acids, and follows the enterohepatic cycle.

Patient Preparation

Patient preparation is essential for proper interpretation. Women must be using contraception or undergo the procedure during the first 10 days of the menstrual cycle; pregnancy is a contraindication. Breast feeding is interrupted. Due to the partial de-iodination of the radiopharmaceutical molecule, thyroid iodine uptake must be blocked by administering excess stable iodine. With NP 59, elimination is predominantly intestinal (Shapiro, 1983); thus, in order to improve image quality, patients undergo careful intestinal preparation. Blocking the iodocholesterol enterohepatic cycle (in association with laxatives) improves adrenal zone visibility by decreasing intestinal and hepatic background activity (Lynn, 1986). Cholestyramine, a resin which binds bile salts within the intestinal lumen, may be administered orally. It must not be administered within 48 hours following tracer injection, which would decrease circulating levels too quickly, and thereby, adrenocortical uptake. Hypercholesterolaemia, inhibitors of steroid synthesis (Op'DDD, aminogluthetimide...), indomethacine, all decrease radiopharmaceutical uptake, while oestrogens and ACTH increase it.

Scintigraphic Technique

NP 59 is slowly injected intravenously at the usual dose of 37 MBq. One or two acquisitions are performed, between 4 and 7 days following injection (up to 14 days for analogues labelled with ^{75}Se). The tracer rapidly binds the adrenal cortex, but late images give a higher signal to background ratio. A wide field camera equipped with a high energy collimator is used. Static images with anterior and posterior incidences are acquired. Single-Photon Emission Computed Tomography (SPECT) has no benefit. The kidneys are localized (using ^{99m}Tc-DTPA) during the initial stages of the exam.

Normal biodistribution

In normal subjects, tracer uptake is observed in both adrenals, usually with low intensity. The right adrenal is deeper than the left. Liver, gall bladder and large intestine may be visualised in case of insufficient preparation.

Indications

This exam may be used in the diagnosis of adrenal mass malignancy. Given the dismal prognosis of ACC, when CT scan criteria do not provide a firm diagnosis orientation, NP 59 scintigraphy may be used to have further information. A qualitative visual interpretation of the exam must be made, knowing the results of endocrine and morphological evaluations.

Adrenal incidentalomas

Adrenal incidentalomas are tumors fortuitously discovered during a morphological examination performed for "non adrenal" reasons. Scintigraphy contributes to distinguish benign from malignant lesions and hypersecretory lesions.

Adrenal cortical adenomas (ACA) intensely take-up iodocholesterol. ACAs of pre-clinical Cushing's syndrome accumulate the tracer and extinguish the contra-lateral gland (because of inhibited ACTH secretion due to cortisol hypersecretion). In this case, uptake is observed ipsi-lateral to the lesion visualised upon CT scan; this is known as "concordant pattern".

ACCs typically capture too little iodocholesterol to be visible. Uptake is absent ipsilateral to the lesion observed on CT scan; this is known as "discordant pattern" *(figure 1)*.

Malignant and/or destructive tumors of non adrenocortical origin (metastases, phaeochromocytomas, ganglioneuromas, liposarcomas, myelolipomas...) or adrenal pseudo-tumors (granulomatosis, haematomas...) do not accumulate the tracer (Gross, 1993, Kloos, 1995).

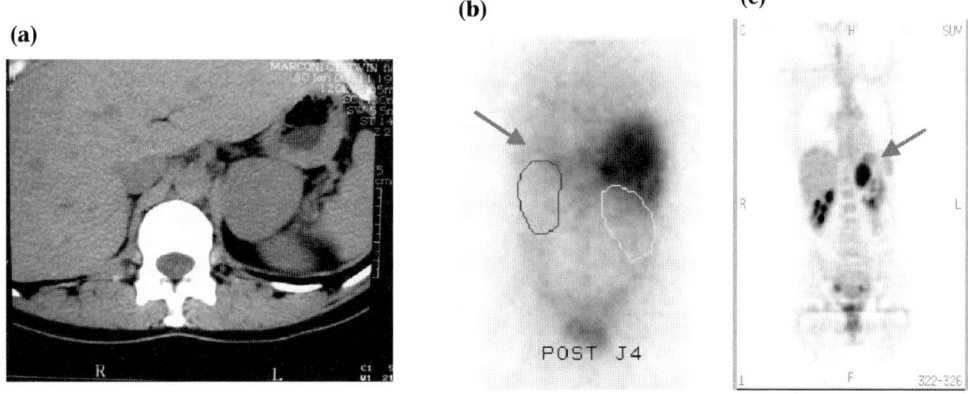

Figure 1. A left ACC:
- (a): A 5 cm tumor with high spontaneous density at CT scan
- (b): "discordant" iodo-cholesterol uptake
- (c): high FDG uptake

For a mass greater than 2 cm, the lack of uptake or the existence of a gap between the usual adrenal uptake and the kidney (localised with ^{99m}Tc DTPA) indicate the extra-adrenal nature of the mass.

For a mass of less than 2 cm, these signs are not valid due to the gamma camera's spatial resolution and the use of iodine 131 (Kloss, 1997).

For the most experienced teams, "concordant pattern" has a 100% accuracy in favour of an adrenocortical adenoma. "Discordant pattern" or the absence of a lateralised uptake anomaly for a mass greater than 2 cm has approximately 100% accuracy in favour of a suspected malignancy (Kloos,1995).

Adrenal Cushing's syndrome

Adrenal Cushing's syndrome is caused by hypersecreting ACA or ACC. ACA typically shows a "concordant pattern" with suppressed contro-lateral uptake. ACCs typically show a bilateral lack of uptake.

The presence of an ACC is suggested by the bilateral non-visualisation of the adrenals: first, as aforementioned, ACC accumulates the tracer poorly, and furthermore, since ACTH secretion is suppressed (under excess cortisol) the normal contro-lateral adrenal gland is not visible. However, rare ACCs are depicted by iodocholesterol, these are highly differentiated, hypersecretory and symptomatic, and do not present as incidentalomas.

Adrenocortical PET (Positron Emission Tomography) with ^{18}F-FDG

Principle

^{18}F-FDG (2-deoxy-2-fluoro-D-glucose labelled with ^{18}F, a positron emitter) is a glucose analogue which competes with glucose at the transmembrane transporter level. In the cell, however, it is not metabolised, and thus accumulates. The neoplastic transformation induced by most cancers induces increased glucose transporter synthesis (particularly GLUT 1) and increased glycolytic enzyme activity (particularly hexokinase). These modifications are responsible for increased glycolytic activity within the cells. However, this phenomenon is not specific to malignant tumors. It may be observed in benign lesions (phaeochromocytomas) (Shulkin, 1999) or in inflammatory diseases (sarcoidosis, granulomatosis) (Strauss, 1996; Cook 1999). Although it is non-specific to any malignancy or to any organ, ^{18}F-FDG has the advantage of being available in all PET centers (Positron Emission Tomography).

Patient preparation

Patients must fast and rest for approximately one and a half hour prior to image acquisition. The patient should be relaxed and, if needed, a benzodiazepine should be administered. He/she should be placed in a dimly lit, calm and warm room, to decrease the risk of false positives due to tracer uptake in skeletal muscles or in brown fat. The exam must be delayed following surgery, radiotherapy and chemotherapy to prevent any possible inflammatory phenomenon from interfering with its interpretation and causing false positives. In diabetic patients, proper glycaemic control is desirable in the days preceding, and especially the day of ^{18}F-FDG injection, in order to obtain satisfactory tracer uptake for proper interpretation.

Technique

Positron Emission Tomography (PET) is a nuclear imaging modality which is becoming more and more widely available: it uses cameras which enable good spatial resolution and whole body images. It is frequently linked with X-ray scans, and when corrected for attenuation, quantification measurements are possible.

^{18}F-FDG is injected intravenously and acquisition performed between 40 and 75 minutes afterwards.

This imaging technique has proven to be effective in a wide variety of oncology settings: characterisation of benign/malignant solitary pulmonary nodules, extension work-ups in numerous neoplasias, and in malignant haematological diseases, pre and post-treatment, and residual mass evaluations.

Normal ^{18}F-FDG biodistribution

^{18}F-FDG accumulates physiologically in the brain and, to varying degrees, in the myocardium. Its elimination being urinary, the kidneys, bladder as well as the urethra are also visualised (Cook, 1999). Uptake is moderate in the liver, spleen and intestine. Image fusion with acquisition using hybrid cameras (PET/CT scan) has enabled these physiological uptakes to be well identified.

Recently, with the use of hybrid cameras, the existence of a physiological adrenal ^{18}F-FDG uptake has been demonstrated in a series of patients with Hodgkin's and non-Hodgkin's tumors, diseases which present a less than 5% prevalence of adrenal involvement. The images made during PET acquisition alone showed that 5% of the normal adrenals were visible with ^{18}F-FDG. A second reading was made using the PET image linked with CT scan, which showed that 68% of the normal adrenal glands actually accumulated ^{18}F-FDG (uptake similar to the background activity or slightly greater than the physiological hepatic uptake) (Bagheri, 2004).

Indications

^{18}F-FDG PET has not yet been validated in differentiating between benign and malignant adrenal masses, contrary to pulmonary nodules (Gould, 2001). However, few studies have examined the role of ^{18}F-FDG PET in the assessment of adrenal masses in oncology patients and for extension work-up of known ACC.

Adrenal masses

The initial data in the exploration of adrenocortical tumors is derived from series of oncology patients. ^{18}F-FDG was performed in extension evaluations, most often in patients with lung cancers (Boland, 1995; Erasmus, 1997; Yun 2001). ^{18}F-FDG correctly classified adrenal metastases: the final diagnosis being made upon biopsy or an increasing mass CT scan at follow-up. An adrenal mass which accumulated ^{18}F-FDG was linked with malignancy (in this case, a metastasis) and an adrenal mass which did not was qualified as benign. Negative ^{18}F-FDG had a high negative predictive value (>95%) in the diagnosis of adrenal metastases from lung cancers.

However, false positives with a normal adrenal biopsy have been described (Erasmus, 1997): the authors note a less intense ^{18}F-FDG uptake in this type of lesion than in metastases.

Concerning adrenal incidentalomas, Maurea *et al.*, 2001 studied non-hypersecretory masses detected upon CT scan or MRI. These included 6 adenomas, 7 benign non-adenoma lesions including 1 phaeochromocytoma, and 13 malignant lesions (metastases, ACCs, sarcomas). The results showed very good sensitivity (100%) and specificity (93% – the phaeochromocytomas accumulated ^{18}F-FDG which is known). The PET scan also participated in extension evaluation by detecting extra-adrenal foci. In an initial preliminary study of 13 patients operated for hypersecretory or non-hypersecretory adrenal masses, excluding a priori adrenal metastases, Tenenbaum *et al.*, 2004 found that 9 out of 9 adenomas did not accumulate ^{18}F-FDG, 3 of 3 ACCs accumulated ^{18}F-FDG and one secondary tumor proved to be an unexpected adrenal metastasis.

Some reports, however, describe occasional benign masses which accumulate ^{18}F-FDG: one adrenocortical adenoma with a pre-clinical Cushing's syndrome (Shimizu, 2003), one adrenocortical adenoma with an adrenal insufficiency with a suspected pre-clinical Cushing's syndrome (Rao, 2004), one myelolipoma (Ludwig, 2002) and one case of bilateral adrenal hyperplasia with a moderate ^{18}F-FDG uptake (Lin, 2002).

Visual interpretation of adrenal ^{18}F-FDG uptake has some limitation when assessing the benign or malignant nature of an adrenal mass. PET/CT scan cameras may be of assistance for the shape and size; uptake intensity may also be measured (SUV: standard uptake value). However, despite these technical improvements, some benign tumors do accumulate ^{18}F-FDG and the origin of this uptake remains incompletely understood.

An ongoing multicentric study is underway at Cochin Hospital to evaluate and compare ^{18}F-FDG-PET with other known means of imaging (CT scan and iodocholesterol scintigraphy) in hypersecretory and non-hypersecretory adrenal tumors, excluding metastases and phaeochromocytomas. All tumors are operated and thus all have a definite pathological diagnosis, including the Weiss score. Currently, out of 50 patients operated for an adrenal mass, 31 were adenomas, 2 of which showed ^{18}F-FDG uptake, 19 were ACCs, all except one necrotic tumor had ^{18}F-FDG uptake (unpublished personal data). ^{18}F-FDG provided additional data in 3 patients revealing unknown metastases sites.

From these preliminary results, it seems that ^{18}F-FDG uptake distinguishes between benign and malignant tumors of the adrenal, and participates in the detection of metastases, and thus in stage classification of the tumor *(figures 2 and 3)*.

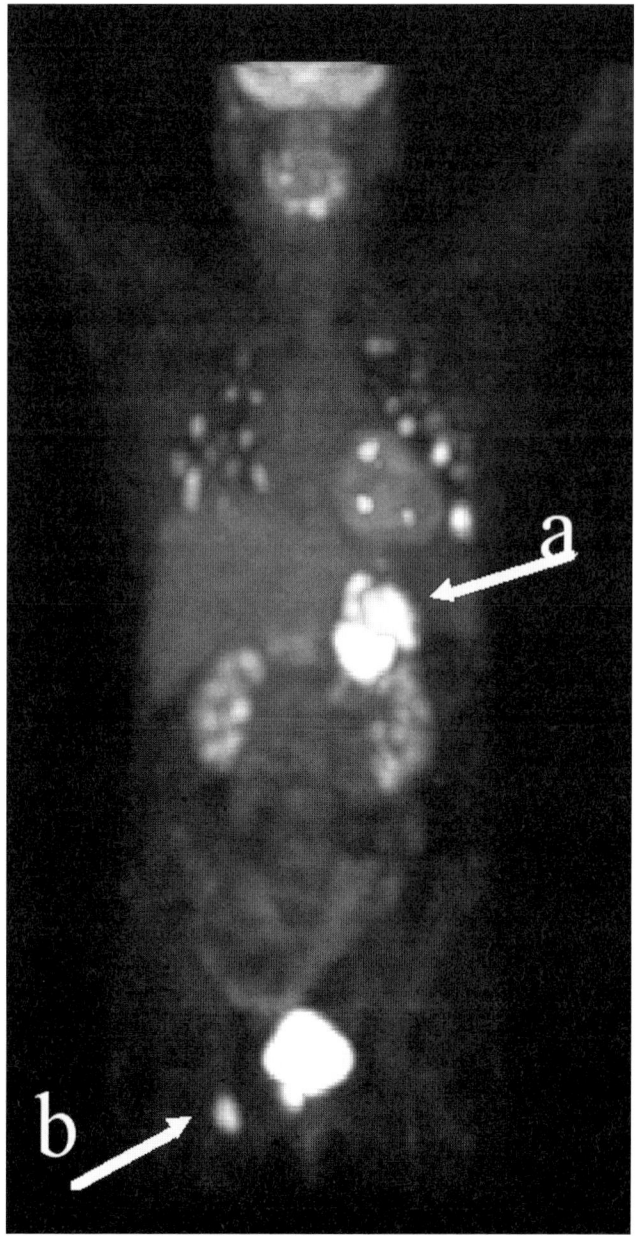

Figure 2. FDG PET in Cushing's syndrome with left ACC (a) and pulmonary metastases. Only FDG PET shows pelvic bone metastases (b).

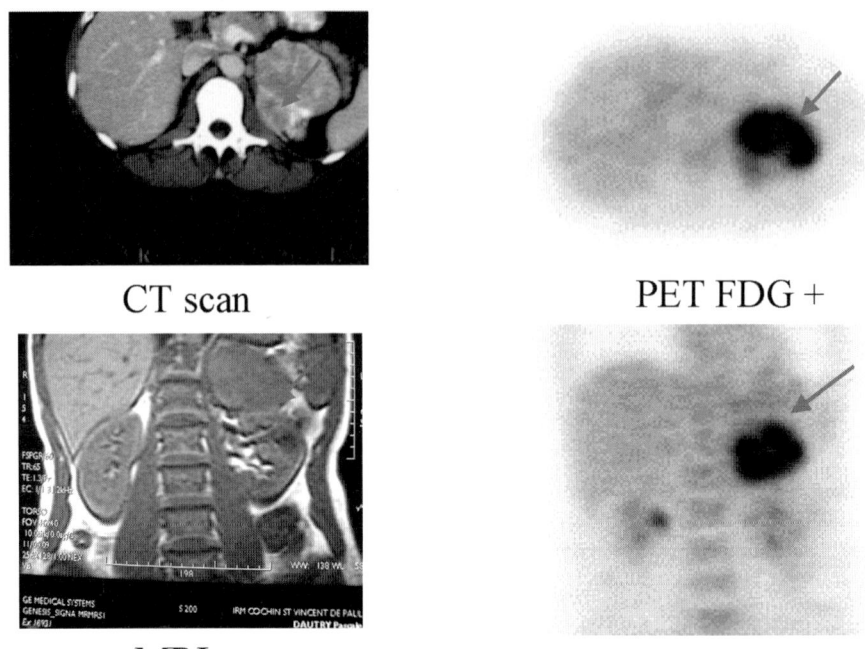

Figure 3. Cushing's syndrome and adrenal tumor (10 cm) corresponding to an ACC. Imaging with CT scan and MRI (left), and FDG PET scan (right).

However, 2 hypersecretory tumors which accumulated ^{18}F-FDG had a Weiss score of 2 and were considered benign. Yet, recent studies have shown that many tumors with a Weiss score of 2 already show an increased prevalence of genetic abnormalities that are associated with a malignant phenotype (loss of heterozygocity at 17p13, at 11p15, IGFII over-expression) (Gicquel, 2001) (see chapter by Bertagna X.).

Thus, it might well be that ^{18}F-FDG PET uptake may yield early information in vivo.

Extension, Evaluation and Adrenal Cortical Carcinoma Surveillance

Concerning ACCs, little data is currently available. Becherer *et al.*, 2001 report on 10 adult patients, studied at the time of diagnosis or during follow-up, comparing ^{18}F-FDG with CT scan and echography. All known sites accumulated ^{18}F-FDG. In three patients, new sites were revealed generating new staging. Op'DDD did not seem to modify ^{18}F-FDG uptake.

A recent study of 28 patients with ACCs (19 known metastatic and 9 considered to be in complete remission) is particularly interesting in terms of comparative imaging (Leboulleux, 2005). Data from PET coupled with ^{18}F-FDG CT scan were compared with data from CT scan alone (thorax, abdomen pelvis), performed within an average delay of 16 days. The study included an analysis per patient, per organ and per lesion in this essentially metastatic series: PET/CT scan with ^{18}F-FDG and CT scan alone have comparable sensitivities (90% and 88% respectively), but these exams are complementary, since 12% and 10%

were visualised by ^{18}F-FDG alone and by CT scan alone respectively. Of particular interest is the detection of local relapses by ^{18}F-FDG (38% visible by ^{18}F-FDG and without CT scan anomalies). Even more interesting, a therapeutic readjustment was possible in some of these cases. The two other noteworthy results from this study were that the tumor size and the mitotic index were significantly correlated with ^{18}F-FDG uptake: high ^{18}F-FDG uptake intensity and tumor volume being poor prognostic factors.

Adrenal cortical examination with a new PET tracer: ^{11}C-metomidate

^{11}C-metomidate is a new radiopharmaceutical specific to the adrenal cortex. Etomidate, utilised as an anaesthetic, is a powerful 11β-hydroxylase inhibitor, a key enzyme in the synthesis of cortisol. Metomidate is an etomidate ester with similar properties; it has been chosen for its synthesis properties. This tracer has strong affinity for the adrenal cortex and the liver, and weak affinity for other organs. Preliminary, results have shown that this tracer is specifically uptaken by adrenocortical lesions, but not by lesions of other origins (metastases, cysts, pheochromocytomas, etc.). However, ^{11}C-metomidate seems to be unable to distinguish between benign and malignant adrenocortical lesions (Bergstrom, 2000; Hennings, 2006).

Conclusion

Currently, scintigraphy with iodocholesterol (NP59), an adrenotropic tracer, remains interesting in diagnosing adrenal mass malignancy. Ongoing studies show that PET with ^{18}F-FDG is a useful means to distinguish between benign and malignant adrenocortical tumors in pre-operative differentiation. It is also useful in adrenal cortical carcinoma extension evaluations, not only to evaluate the number of sites, but also to determine patient prognosis. In addition, this exam seems to be particularly important in the detection of local relapses.

A new PET radiopharmaceutical (^{11}C-metomidate, a 11β-hydroxylase inhibitor specific to the adrenal cortex) is under evaluation.

References

Bagheri B, Maurer AH, Cone L, Doss L, Adler L. Characterization of the normal adrenal gland with 18F-FDG PET/CT. *J Nucl Med* 2004; 45: 1340.

Becherer A, Vierhapper H, Potzi C, Karanikas G, Kurturan A, Schmaljohann J. FDG-PET in adrenocortical carcinoma Cancer. *Biother Radiopharm* 2001; 16: 289-95.

Beierwaltes WH, Wieland DM, Yu T, Swanson D, Mosley S. Adrenal imaging agents: rationale, synthesis, formulation and metabolism. *Seminars in Nuclear Medicine* 1978; 8: 5-21.

Bergström M, Juhlin C, Bonasera TA, Sundin A, Rastad J, Akerstrom G, Langstrom B. PET imaging of adrenal cortical tumors with the 11beta-hydroxylase tracer 11C-metomidate. *J Nucl Med* 2000; 41: 275-82.

Boland GW, Goldberg MA, Lee MJ, Mayo-Smith WW, Dixon J, McNicholas MM, et al. Indeterminate adrenal mass in patients with cancer: evaluation at PET with 2-(F-18)-fluoro-2deoxy-D-glucose. *Radiology* 1995; 194: 131-4.

Cook GJ, Maisey MN, Fogelman I. Normal variants, artifacts and interpretative pitfalls in PET imaging with 18-fluoro-2-deoxy-glucose and carbone-11 methionine. *Eur J Nucl Med* 1999; 26: 1363-78.

Erasmus JJ, Patz EF, McAdams HP, Murray JC, Herndon J, Coleman RE, et al. Evaluation of adrenal masses in patients with bronchogenic carcinoma using 18F-fluorodeoxyglucose positron emission tomography. *Am J Roentgenol* 1997; 168: 1357-60.

Gicquel C, Bertagna X, Gaston V, Coste J, Louvel A, Baudin E, et al. Molecular markers and long-term recurrences in a large cohort of patients with sporadic adrenocortical tumors. *Cancer Res* 2001; 61: 6762-7.

Gould MK, Maclean CC, Kuschner WG, Rydazk CE, Owen DK. Accuracy of positron emission tomography for diagnosis of pulmonary nodules and mass lesions: a meta-analysis. *Journal of the American Medical Association* 2001; 285: 914-24.

Gross MD, Shapiro B. Clinical review: clinically silent adrenal masses. *J Clin Endocrinol Metab* 1993; 77: 885-8.

Hennings J, Lindhe O, Bergström M, Sundin A, Hellman P. 11C-metomidate positron emission tomography of adrenocortical tumors in correlation with histopathological findings. *J Clin Endocrinol Metabol* 2006; jan (10).

Kloos RT, Gross MD, Francis IR, Korobkin M, Shapiro B. Incidentally discovered adrenal masses. *Endocrine Reviews* 1995; 16: 460-84.

Kloos RT, Gross MD, Shapiro B, Francis IR, Korobkin M, Thompson NW. Diagnostic dilemma of small incidentally discovered adrenal masses: role for 131I-6?-iodomethyl-norcholesterol scintigraphy. *World J Surg* 1997; 21: 36-40.

Leboulleux S, Dromain C, Bonniaud G, Auperin A, Caillou B, Lumbroso J, et al. Diagnostic and prognostic value of 18-fluorodeoxyglucose positron emission tomography in adrenocortical carcinoma: a prospective comparison with computed tomography. *J Clin Endocrinol Metabol* 2006; 91: 926-32.

Lin EC, Helgans R. Adrenal hyperplasia in Cushing's syndrome demonstrated by FDG positron emission tomographic imaging. *Clin Nucl Med* 2002; 27: 516-7.

Ludwig V, Rice MH, Martin WH, Kelley MC, Delbeke D. 2-Deoxy-2-[18F]fluoro-D-glucose positron emission tomography uptake in a giant adrenal myelolipoma. *Mol Imaging Biol* 2002; 4: 355-8.

Lynn MD, Gross MD, Shapiro B. Enterohepatic circulation and distribution of 131-I-6-iodomethyl-19-norcholesterol (NP-59). *Nucl Med Commun* 1986; 7: 625-30.

Maurea S, Klain M, Mainolfi C, Ziviello M, Salvatore M. The diagnostic of radionuclide imaging in evaluation of patients with nonhypersecreting adrenal masses. *J Nucl Med* 2001; 42: 884-92.

Rao SK, Caride VJ, Ponn R, Giakovis E, Lee SH. F-18 fluorodeoxyglucose positron emission tomography-positive benign adrenal cortical adenoma: imaging features and pathologic correlation. *Clin Nucl Med* 2004; 29: 300-2.

Sarkar SD, Cohen EL, Beierwaltes WH, Ice RD, Cooper R, Gold EN. A new and superior adrenal imaging agent 131I-6Biodomethyl-19-nor-cholesterol (NP-59): evaluation in humans. *J Clin Endocrinol Metab* 1977; 45: 353-62.

Shapiro B, Britton KE, Hawkins LA, Edwards CE. Clinical experience with 75-Se-selenomethylcholesterol adrenal imaging. *Clinical Endocrinology* 1981; 15: 19-27.

Shapiro B, Nakajo M, Gross MD, et al. Value of bowel preparation in adrenocortical scintigraphy with NP-59. *J Nucl Med* 1983; 24: 732-4.

Shimizu A, Oriuchi N, Tsushima Y, Higuchi T, Aoki J, Endo K. High (18F) 2-fluoro-2-deoxy-D-glucose (FDG) uptake of adrenocortical adenoma showing subclinical Cushing's syndrome. *Ann Nucl Med* 2003; 17: 403-6.

Shulkin BL, Thompson NW, Shapiro B, Francis IR, Sisson JC. Pheochromocytomas: imaging with 2-fluorine-18-fluoro-2deoxy-D-glucose PET. *Radiology* 1999; 212: 35-41.

Strauss LG. Fluorine-18 deoxyglucose and false-positive results: a major problem in diagnosis of oncological patients. *Eur J Nucl Med* 1996; 23: 1409-15.

Tenenbaum F, Groussin L, Foehrenbach H, Tissier F, Gouya H, Bertherat J. *et al.* 18F-fluorodeoxyglucose positron emission tomography as a diagnostic tool for malignancy of adrenocortical tumors? Preliminary results in 13 consecutive patients. *Eur J Endocrinol* 2004; 150: 789-92.

Yun M, Kim W, Alnafisi N, Lacorte L, Jang S, Alavi A. 18F-FDGPET in characterizing adrenal lesions detected on CT or MRI. *J Nucl Med* 2001; 42: 1795-9.

Adrenal cortical tumors in childhood

Cécile Thomas-Teinturier, Pierre-François Bougnères
Paediatric Endocrinology Department, Saint Vincent de Paul Hospital, Faculty of Medicine René Descartes, Univ. Paris 5

Adrenal cortical neoplasm is rare in childhood, with adrenal cortical carcinomas accounting for the majority of these tumors (80-90%). They have some typical characteristics in infancy. These characteristics concern epidemiologic data, genetic predisposition, histology, clinical and hormonal presentation and a definite better prognosis than in adults.

Epidemiology of paediatric adrenal cortical tumors

Adrenal cortical tumors are rare in children, with an incidence of 0.3 per million children below 15 years (Stiller, 1994). While neuroblastoma represents over 90% of adrenal tumors in childhood, adrenal cortical carcinoma accounts for only 6% of these tumors. It constitutes 0.2% of all childhood cancers (Bernstein, 1999).

In the state of Parana, southern Brazil, adrenal cortical carcinoma is as high as 3.4 per million children, a figure 15 times greater than that in other geographic regions (Sandrini, 1997). The reason for this was unclear until a few years ago, when Ribeiro reported that these children had in common a unique constitutional mutation of the p53 gene, which predisposes to this cancer (see genetics).

The Surveillance Epidemiology End Results data indicate about 14 new cases per year in individuals younger than age 20 years in the United States.

Genetic predisposition

Adrenal cortical carcinoma in childhood is frequently associated with a genetic predisposition. Two syndromes are well recognized as associated with this condition, Beckwith-Wiedemann syndrome or hemihypertrophy, and Li-Fraumeni syndrome.

Hemihypertrophy and Beckwith-Wiedemann syndrome

Beckwith-Wiedemann syndrome and hemihypertrophy are overgrowth disorders caused in more than 70% of cases by dysfunction of the expression of imprinted genes in the 11p15 chromosomal locus. Molecular diagnosis is currently difficult, mostly due to the large spectrum of genetic and epigenetic abnormalities. This syndrome causes a complex cancer-susceptibility disorder, associated with other abnormalities. Beckwith-Wiedemann syndrome was first described in 1964 and is characterised by omphalocele, macroglossia, macrosomia, neonatal hypoglycaemia, ear pits or ear creases and midline abdominal wall-defects (Wiedemann, 1964). The estimated frequency of this disorder is 1 in 13700 newborns. Hemihypertrophy may be a partial form of the same syndrome (figure 1). Its incidence is estimated to be 1/86000 live birth. Children with these syndromes are at increased risk of malignant and benign tumors, including Wilms' tumor, adrenal cortical tumors, hepatoblastoma, neuroblastoma and rhabdomyosarcoma. Adrenal cortical

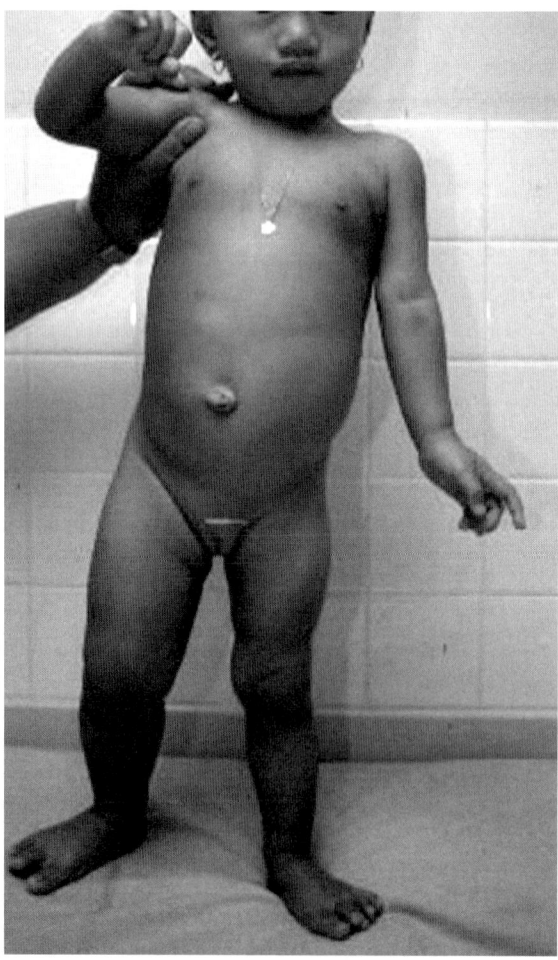

Figure 1. Hemihypertrophy of the right leg and abdominal mass in a 13 months old girl.

tumor is the second most common tumor in these syndromes (15-20% of patients) (Hoyme, 1998; Wiedemann 1983).

Li-Fraumeni syndrome

Li and Fraumeni observed a remarkably high frequency of adrenal cortical tumors (10%) among 44 malignancies in children from families in which diverse cancers segregated in an autosomal dominant pattern (Li, 1988). In 1990, Malkin *et al.* screened these families and found germline mutations in exon 7 of the p53 gene. These p53 gene abnormalities predispose to numerous cancers, of the breast, the brain, soft tissue sarcomas and osteosarcomas, leukaemia and adrenal cortical carcinoma, occurring before the age of 45 years. It is now well recognised that most of the constitutional genetic abnormalities in young children with adrenal cortical tumors are germline mutations in various exons of the p53 gene. They have been found in 9 of 13 cases of paediatric adrenal cortical tumors selected without reference to the family's history of cancer (Varley, 1999). In southern Brazil, a unique constitutional p53 mutation (R337H) is found in 35/36 children with adrenal cortical carcinoma before the age of 4 years. In these cases, the families have had an unremarkable cancer history (Ribeiro, 2001). An evolving hypothesis is that this p53 mutation has low penetrance for cancer susceptibility in general, but is associated with a specific increased predisposition to paediatric adrenal cortical carcinomas. The biological basis of this finding has only now begun to be elucidated. This Arg 337 to His mutation is in the tetramerization domain of p53 and results in a mutant, which is less stable than the wild type and highly sensitive to pH in the physiological range (DiGiammarino, 2002). Older children and young adults with adrenal cortical tumors rarely carry this germline p53 mutation; only 13% of a Brazilian population with adrenocortical tumor does (Latronico, 2001). Patients from other countries have rarely been tested for p53 abnormalities. But these have been found in 45-70% of children with adrenocortical carcinoma, although it was never the specific mutation that was identified in the Brazilian patients. It is plausible that the presence of a constitutional p53 mutation increases the penetrance of adrenal cortical tumors in the foetal adrenal cortex but not in the definite adrenal cortex. This premise is consistent with the fact that in individuals with constitutional p53 mutations, adrenal cortical tumors usually occur only during the first decade of life (Kleihues, 1997).

Pathology

One of the facts about adrenal cortical tumors in childhood is that an adrenal cortical neoplasm may have pathologic features, more often of a microscopic nature, that by all other conventions qualify for an interpretation of malignancy, but whose prognosis is otherwise durable disease-free interval and often definitive cure after complete surgical resection. The behaviour of these lesions can be quite distinct from their histological similar counterparts in the adult population, making pathologic criteria for distinguishing benign from malignant tumors equivocal. The established criteria for distinguishing benign from malignant adrenal cortical tumors in the adult population have not been helpful in predicting the behaviour of such neoplasm in children (Weiss, 1989; Medeiros, 1992; Hawkins, 1992). On the basis of pathologic criteria used in adults, 80-90% of adrenal cortical tumors in children are carcinomas. However, the prognosis of adrenal cortical carcinoma in children is clearly more favourable when compared with adults. A clinical pathologic study of 83 adrenal cortical tumors presenting in the first two decades of life brings some clarity on this subject (Wieneke, 2003). The focus of the study was pathologic discrimination between a group of tumors histologically malignant and clinically benign and another group histological and clinically malignant tumors. In multivariate analysis, only the presence of necrosis alone or the presence of increased mitotic activity alone (based on > 15/20 HPF) increased the likelihood of malignant behaviour ($p = 0.05$ and $p = 0.002$ respectively). The presence of nuclear hyperchromasia and microcalcifications, although not statistically significant, is only seen in histological malignant cases. But none of these features can be used solely as a predictor of malignancy: necrosis, for example, is present in half of the children with a good clinical outcome. Therefore, it is important to stress that no single histological feature is diagnostic for malignancy; a constellation of histomorphologic features must be taken into account for a diagnosis of adrenal cortical carcinoma in children. *Tables I and II* show the nine pathologic features of malignancy and the correlation between the number of these features in a neoplasm and clinical outcome. Three or less unfavourable pathologic features would appear to be the breakpoint or threshold between clinically benign and malignant adrenocortical tumors. We must keep in mind that there is a significant overlap in histological features between paediatric carcinomas with a good clinical outcome and those with poor outcome *(tables I, II)*. It is worth noting, in light of the adult criteria, that the following features had no significant impact on patient outcome: severe nuclear pleomorphism, broad fibrous band and predominance of lipid-poor, compact cells with eosinophilic cytoplasm (Wieneke, 2003).

Table I. Proposed criteria for malignancy of adrenocortical neoplasms in paediatric patients (from Wieneke, 2003).

Tumor weight > 400 g
Tumor size > 10.5 cm
Extension into periadrenal soft tissues and/or adjacent organs
Invasion into vena cava
Venous invasion
Capsular invasion
Presence of tumor necrosis
> 15 mitoses per 20 HPF (high-power field (400x)
Presence of atypical mitotic figures

Table II. Separating clinically benign from clinically malignant paediatric adrenal cortical neoplasms (from Wieneke, 2003).

Cumulative number of criteria present*	Number of clinically benign cases	Number of clinically malignant cases
0	10	0
1	17	2
2	8	0
3	15	3
4	5	3
5	2	4
6	2	5
7	1	5
8	0	0
9	0	1

* Criteria as listed in *table I*

Disease staging

Disease staging criteria for childhood adrenal cortical tumors generally have not been agreed upon. Most investigators use a classification scheme proposed by Mac Farlane and modified by Sullivan. This classification, which is based on tumor size, lymph node involvement, local invasiveness and metastatic disease, has been developed for adults. For children, Sandrini proposed a modification of this staging system *(table III)* (Sandrini, 1997). These modifications are based on the premise that complete tumor resection and tumor size are the most important factors for disease control. These criteria allowed the identification of 3 distinctive prognostic groups. Patients with completely resected small tumors (< 200 cm^3 or 6 cm in diameter) had an excellent prognosis, whereas patients with either microscopic or gross residual disease had a poor prognosis. The prognostic accuracy of this classification for the intermediate groups can probably be improved by adding information on pathology, lymph node invasion, capsular rupture during surgery and tumor biological markers.

Molecular markers in paediatric tumors

Genetic or epigenetic alterations of chromosomal region 11p15 (allelic loss, paternal isodisomy, loss of imprinting and overexpression of the insulin-like growth factor II gene) are constantly found in paediatric adrenal cortical tumors, indicating involvement of 11p15 region dysfunction in the early stages of adrenal tumorigenesis in childhood (Henry, 1989; Gicquel, 2002; Wilkin, 2000).

Allelic loss at the 17p13 locus occurs in 50-60% of adrenal cortical tumors in children, compared to 38% of such tumors in adults (Gicquel, 2001). Whether this chromosome 17 loss correlates with tumor aggressiveness in paediatric adrenal cortical tumors is still controversial. In the 16 paediatric tumors tested by Gicquel et al, 9 showed 17p13 loss of heterozygosity, 3 stage 4, 5 stage 2 and 1 stage 1 tumor that recurred after the initial surgery. All tumors without this chromosome 17 loss were stage 1 or 2, and none of these patients experienced a relapse. Although the prognostic value of this abnormality cannot be determined precisely, it seems to be associated with more aggressive tumors (Gicquel, 2002). In Brazilian patients, the isolated loss of chromosome 17 did not correlate with aggressive tumor behaviour in 30 adrenal cortical tumors: 16 in children and 14 in adults (Pinto, 2005).

Table III. Modified Disease Staging System for paediatric adrenal cortical tumors.

Stage	Description
I	Tumor completely excised with negative margins, tumor weight < 200g, and absence of metastasis
II	Tumor completely excised with negative margins, tumor weight > 200g, and absence of metastasis
III	Residual* or inoperable tumor
IV	Metastasis

* Residual tumor is defined as the presence of microscopic or gross tumor after surgical resection

Using comparative genomic hybridization, Figueiredo *et al.* have demonstrated a number of chromosomal gains and losses in adrenal cortical tumors in children from southern Brazil (Figueiredo, 1999). The most consistent finding was the presence of copy number gains in chromosomal region 9q34. There were increased copy numbers of the steroidogenic factor 1 (SF-1) gene, which is located in this region and plays an important role in the development and function of the adrenal cortex, suggesting a relationship with adrenocortical tumorigenesis in children (Figueiredo, 2005).

Clinical and hormonal manifestations in children

Because of the rarity of paediatric adrenal cortical tumors, few paediatric departments have acquired extensive experience with this tumor. Most reported series describe only a few patients observed over a period of several years. Analysis of the literature reveals few series describing more than 20 patients, most of them of Brazilian origin (Sabbaga, 1993; Sandrini, 1997; Wieneke, 2003; Michalkiewicz, 2004). Only 4 are European studies (Lefevre, 1983; Wolthers, 1999; Ciftci, 2001; Teinturier, 1999). Liou and Kay summarized the clinical and outcome data for 412 patients from several published series, mostly from the United States (Liou, 2000). Better knowledge of this tumor in childhood is provided by the original report of the 254 patients registered on the International Paediatric Adrenocortical Tumor Registry, 80% of whom come from southern Brazil (Michalkiewicz, 2004). The main clinical characteristics of the patients described in the literature are summarised in *table IV*.

In all published paediatric series, excepted the French one, adrenal cortical tumor is more frequently seen in females. Sex ratio is 1.6 female/1 male. The reason for the predominance of female sex in children with adrenal cortical tumors is not known (just as in adults).

Median age at diagnosis of the tumor is 3 to 4 years. There is a biphasic age distribution, with 50-60% of cases presenting in children under the age of 4 and only 15-20% in children over the age of 13 years *(figure 2)*.

Virilisation alone or in combination with signs of overproduction of other adrenal cortical hormones is the most common clinical presentation (80-90% of patients). The presenting features of virilisation include pubic hair, clitoromegaly or penile enlargement, facial acne, facial hair, hirsutism and growth acceleration *(figures 3, 4)*. Cushing's syndrome is rare (5-20%) and tends to occur in the older children (mean age 12 yrs).

Non-functional tumors are even rarer in the paediatric population, accounting for less than 10% and occurring at a mean age of 6 years.

Hypertension is observed at the time of diagnosis in nearly 50% of patients. In a few patients, it is severe enough to cause encephalopathy. Hypertension is attributed in part to tumor production of either glucocorticoids and/or mineralocorticoids, but it can be due to tumor compression of the renal artery.

Table IV. Clinical characteristics of paediatric adrenocortical tumors reported in the literature.

	N	Sex ratio F/M	Median age (yr)	Virilisation (%)	Cushing's syndrome (%)	Stages I, II (%)	Stage III (%)	Stage IV (%)	5-year Survival
Michalkiewicz	254	1.6/1	3.3	84%	34.5%	75%	9.8%	14.6%	54.7%
Wieneke	83	1.5/1	4	60%	35%		27%		74.7%
Sandrini	58	2.1/1	4.3	90%	53%	78%	7%	15%	30/54
Sabbaga	55	3.2/1		95%	74%			18%	46%
Teinturier	54	1/1	4	76%	15%	78%	9%	13%	49%
Lefevre	42	1.6/1	4	93%	38%				22/42
Wolthers	30	3.2/1	4.9 (mean)	100%*	13%	77%	23%		26/30
Ciftci	30	1.7/1	6.7 (mean)	50%	30%	47%	43%	10%	15/26

* By deliberate choice

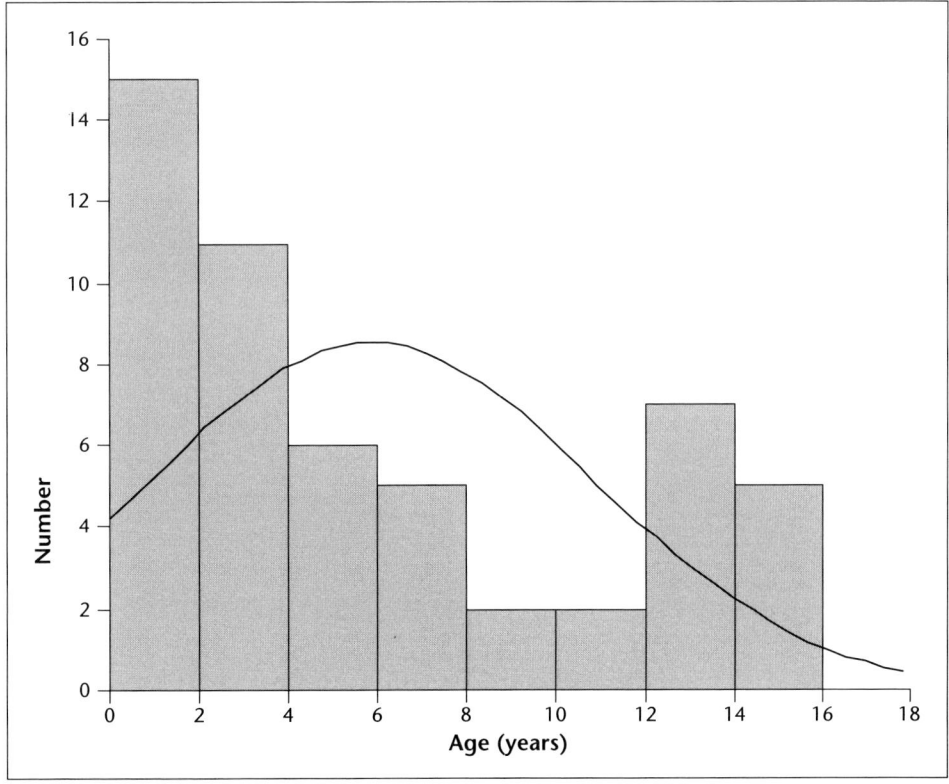

Figure 2. Age distribution of 54 paediatric adrenal cortical tumors (Teinturier, 1999).

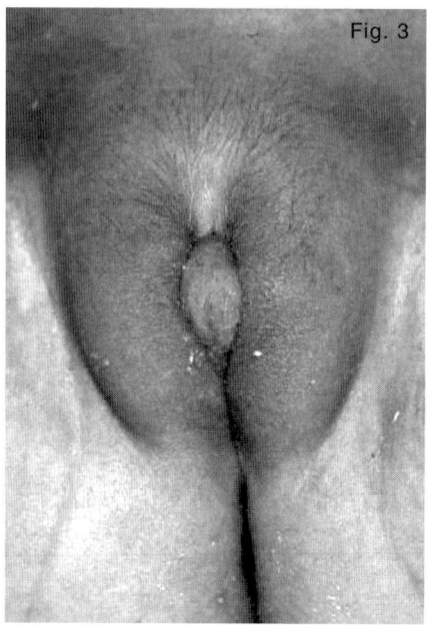

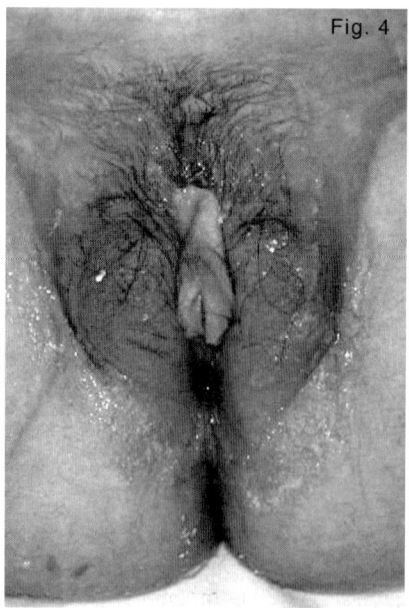

Figures 3 and 4. Symptoms of virilisation due to adrenal cortical carcinoma in 2 girls less than 2 years of age: pubic hair and clitoromegaly.

Most tumors secrete androgens alone (40%), or associated with glucocorticoids (25%), estrogens (18%), or both (11%). High serum concentration of adrenal androgens, especially DHEA-S, 10 to 100 fold above the normal value for age and sex, is highly suggestive of this kind of tumor. Median values and ranges of steroid levels in a French study of paediatric adrenal cortical tumors are shown in *table V*.

More than two thirds of the patients have limited disease: 44% stage I disease and 31% stage II. Among patients with advanced disease, 10% have stage III and 15% have stage IV disease. Sites of metastases are mostly pulmonary and/or hepatic.

The analysis of the data in the literature suggests that paediatric adrenal cortical tumors are heterogeneous, and comprise at least two distinct disease groups according to the age of children. Patients who have a diagnosis within the first 4 years of life tend to be girls. Girls and boys younger than 12 years of age do not differ in clinical and hormonal features or in constitutional p53 mutations in the Brazilian population. However, the clinical presentation seen in the older group differs from that observed in the younger group and is similar to that in adults. Adolescents tend to have Cushing's syndrome or non-functional tumors at presentation and germ line p53 mutations are relatively rare. According to Michalkiewicz, in the young child, the predominance of virilising tumors and their histopathological features suggest that adrenal cortical tumors arise from the foetal zone of the adrenal cortex. The foetal zone represents 85% of the adrenal cortex during foetal development and is oriented toward dehydroepiandrosterone production, as indicated by the fact that the foetal zone cells express enzyme 17a-hydroxylase/17,20 lyase (p450c17) (Keegan, 2002). In contrast, adrenal cortical carcinoma of adolescence and adulthood may originate from the definite adrenal cortex.

Treatment

Surgical treatment has long been the cornerstone of therapy for adrenocortical tumors. It is the only therapy that unquestionably cures or prolongs survival significantly. Therefore, curative surgical resection should be considered for every child with adrenocortical tumors. It is important to remember that these patients need perioperative steroid coverage. Total resection is necessary and needs a transabdominal approach. Because of extensive tumor necrosis, haemorrhage and fibrosis, these tumors are particularly friable and are susceptible to intraoperative tumor rupture and spillage.

Spontaneous tumor rupture and tumor rupture after percutaneous biopsies have also been reported. Therefore, needle biopsy should be avoided in children with adrenal cortical tumor. Before tumor resection, the inferior vena cava and the controlateral adrenal should always be palpated to detect thrombus or bilateral tumor that can be extracted during the initial surgery. The laparoscopic method should be avoided in the management for paediatric adrenal cortical tumors because it can lead to tumor rupture and seeding during the procedure, and to subsequent relapse. The role of regional lymphnode dissection in paediatric adrenal cortical tumors has not been evaluated, and the recommendation is to widely sample the lymph nodes and to proceed with radical lymph node dissection when the biopsy is positive.

Surgical resection should also be considered for solitary metastases and locally recurrent tumor.

The efficacy of chemotherapy in adrenal cortical tumors in children is still under evaluation. O,p'DDD, an isomer of the insecticide p,p'DDD, specifically induces adrenocortical necrosis. O,p'DDD has been used to treat advanced or metastatic adrenal cortical tumors prior to surgery in cases of inoperable tumors, or after curative surgery in children at high risk of relapse (adjuvant therapy). Its role as adjuvant therapy is still controversial. Response rates, about 30%, appears to be similar to that seen in adults (Lefevre, 1983; Mayer, 1997; Teinturier, 1999). Significant reduction of large tumors allowing surgical resection, as well as regression of metastases with definitive cure, have been reported in children (Teinturier, 1999; Godil, 2000; De Leon, 2002). But this drug has significant toxicity, affecting mostly the gastrointestinal, neurological and endocrine system in children. Inadequate control of O,p'DDD inducing adrenal insufficiency may even lead to death in infants (Teinturier, 1999). All patients receiving this agent should be considered to have severe adrenal insufficiency and need careful medical supervision, with adjustment of the dosage of hydrocortisone and fludrocortisone during episodes of infection.

There has been no formal trial of conventional chemotherapy agents in paediatric adrenal cortical tumors, but the available case reports suggest that a subset of this tumor is chemotherapy sensitive. The combination used most often in children consists of Cisplatinum or Carboplatinum and Etoposide given in conjunction with O,p'DDD. Some anecdotal observations report long term survival after treatment of metastatic adrenal cortical tumors with this combination, but most of the patients relapse after discontinuation of chemotherapy (Crock, 1989; Ayass, 1991; Teinturier, 1999). Systematic studies to determine the overall rate of response to this combination chemotherapy are needed.

Other adjunctive therapeutic modalities, such as radiotherapy can be effective in some cases, but they have not been well studied in children (Lefevre, 1983).

Outcome and prognostic factors

Prognosis of adrenal cortical tumors is better in children than in adults. Children with histological malignant-appearing adrenal cortical tumor often do better than their adult counterparts. The 5-year overall survival estimates are 46-68%, with 5-year event free survival estimates of 46-64% *(table IV)*. Approximately 70% of children with histological malignant-appearing tumor have a benign clinical course without recurrence (Wieneke, 2003). After a 5-year follow-up, the risk of developing recurrence diminishes dramatically. Because surgery is the only known effective treatment for this tumor, complete tumor resection is the single most important prognostic factor. Long term survival rate is around 70-75% for children with completely resected tumors, and only 7-14% for those who have distant or local gross or microscopic residual disease after surgery (Teinturier, 1999; Michalkiewicz, 2004).

This raises the question: are there any criteria that one can use to predict the biologic behaviour of completely excised adrenal cortical neoplasm in paediatric patients in order to guide therapeutic management decisions?

Tumor size and tumor weight correlate with patient outcome, thus a tumor size > 10 cm or a tumor weight > 400 g suggest a poor outcome. Inversely, weight < 200 g identifies a group of patients with very good prognosis. But this did not prove to be an independent prognostic factor and so cannot be used as the sole criterion for malignancy. Several children in the literature have been reported with large tumors and yet enjoyed a good clinical outcome, whereas small tumors yielded a malignant outcome in others. Although girls are more frequently affected than boys, gender has not proven to be a statistically significant prognostic factor. Age younger than 4 years seems to be independently associated with a better survival in a multivariate analysis based on the largest study published (Michalkiewicz, 2004). And, in some series, the adolescent group tends to have a worse prognosis. Whereas a functional tumor may be indicative of poor outcome in adult patients, the same cannot be extrapolated to the paediatric population. By contrast, virilisation as the sole clinical manifestation is associated with better prognosis. Other features are found to be statistically predictive of worse patient outcome: Cushing's syndrome, extension into periadrenal soft tissues and/or adjacent organs, rupture of the tumor pseudocapsule during surgery and invasion into the vena cava.

Some authors attempted to separate the carcinomas with good and poor outcome based on the number of criteria present *(table I)*. It is important in a grading system not to undertreat a potentially malignant tumor, and not to overtreat those with a good clinical outcome. Therefore, there is no clear breakpoint above or below which patients can be accurately classified *(table II)*. However, several factors have been identified, which when aggregated, appear to accurately predict a more aggressive behaviour *(table I)*. As more features are seen, a trend toward malignant

Table V. Mean values and ranges of steroid levels in children with secreting adrenal cortical tumors (from Teinturier, 1999).

	Mean ± SE	Range	Normal range*
Androgens			
DHA (ng/ml): (n = 26)	13.6 ± 2	1.7 – 33	0.05 – 2
DHAS (ng/ml): (n = 23)	9773 ± 2178	470 – 48800	48 – 320
Androstenedione (ng/ml): (n = 27)	6.2 ± 1.5	1.6 – 35	< 0.05 – 0.45
Testosterone (ng/ml): (n = 31)	20.9 ± 19.7	0.15 – 543	< 0.05 – 0.20
17-ketosteroids (mg/d): (n = 35)	88 ± 22	2 – 415	< 3
Estrogens			
Estradiol-17 ß (pg/ml) (n = 16)	64 ± 13	15 – 302	< 5 – 20
Estrone (pg/ml) (n = 13)	88 ± 27	17 – 511	< 8 – 35
Glucocorticoïds			
Free urinary cortisol (µg/d) (n = 11)	435 ± 95	38 – 1670	< 35
17-hydroxycorticosteroids (mg/d) (n = 9)	19 ± 2.6	10 – 50	< 3

* Normal values from our laboratory (Dr. N. Lahlou) for girls 5 to 8 years old

behaviour is definitely identified. But no clear separation is now known that could provide a valuable indication in the prospective management of patients. A specific number of pathologic criteria in no way guarantees the development of metastatic disease nor dictates that the patient will die from his disease. Neither does a specific number guarantee a benign outcome.

Treatment options and strategies

In summary, children aged less than 4 years old, with localized, small (< 5-10 cm in their largest diameter or < 100-200g), only virilising and with completely excised tumor have an excellent prognosis and require no further treatment. The expected relapse rate is less than 10%.

At the other extreme are patients with residual or metastatic tumor who need multimodality therapy with surgery and chemotherapy.

Between the two, are patients who have completely resected tumor but are at high risk of relapse (adolescent with Cushing's syndrome, loco-regional disease and histopathological poor prognostic factors). O,p'DDD given alone as adjuvant therapy in these patients in order to prevent recurrence during one or two years after surgery must be proposed but has not been adequately evaluated in children.

There is a small group of patients who have a very large abdominal mass without metastases, which cannot be safely resected. For these patients, O,p'DDD is recommended to induce tumor shrinkage and improve the odds of secondarily complete resection.

Finally, there is an intermediate or indeterminate group of patients who needs to have clinical follow-up similar to those that are frank carcinomas, at least until a 5-year period is achieved to exclude a recurrence.

Conclusion

Adrenal cortical carcinoma in younger children, whose pathologic counterpart is lethal in adults, is seemingly a fundamentally different disease in terms of its clinical presentation and behaviour. As the age at diagnosis of an adrenocortical carcinoma approaches adulthood, so the prognosis tends towards the poorer outcome associated with this neoplasm in older individuals.

Despite the number of recent studies on the molecular biology of adrenocortical tumors, there are still many unanswered questions about a neoplasm that has the potential for spontaneous regression of metastatic disease in an infant, yet is a consistently lethal neoplasm in an adult (Saracco, 1988; Kasat, 2001).

References

Ayass M, Gross S, Harper J. High-dose carboplatinum and VP16 in treatment of metastatic adrenal carcinoma. *Am J Pediatr Hematol Oncol* 1991; 13: 470-2.

Bernstein L, Gurney JG. Carcinomas and other malignant epithelial neoplasms. In: Ries LAG, Smith MA, Gurney JG, et al., eds. Cancer incidence and survival among children and adolescents: United States SEER program 1975 1995. Bethesda, MD, National Cancer Institute, SEER program, 1999, 139-147.

Crock PA, Clark ACL. Combination chemotherapy for adrenal carcinoma: Response in a 5 1/2-year-old-male. *Med Pediatr Oncol* 1989; 17: 62-5.

Ciftci AO, Senocak ME, Tanyel FC. Adrenal cortical tumors in children. *J Pediatr Surg* 2001; 36: 549-54.

De Leon DD, Lange BJ, Walterhouse D, Moshang T. Long term (15 years) outcome in an infant with metastatic adrenocortical carcinoma. *J Clin Endocrinol Metab* 2002; 87: 4452-6.

DiGiammarino EL, Lee AS, Cadwell C, Zhang W, Bothner B, Ribeiro RC, et al. A novel mechanism of tumorigenesis involving pH-dependent destabilization of a mutant p53 tetramer. *Nat struct Biol* 2002; 9: 12-6.

Figueiredo BC, Stratakis CA, Sandrini R, DeLacerda L, Pianovsky MA, Giatzakis C, et al. Comparative genomic hybridization analysis of adrenocortical tumors of childhood. *J Clin Endocrinol Metab* 1999, 84: 1116-21.

Figueiredo BC, Cavalli LR, Pianovsky MA, Lalli E, Sandrini R, Ribeiro RC, et al. Amplification of the steroidogenic factor 1 gene in childhood adrenocortical tumors. *J Clin Endocrinol Metab* 2005; 90: 615-9.

Gicquel C, Bertagna X, Gaston V, Coste J, Louvel A, Baudin E, et al. Molecular markers and long-term recurrences in a large cohort of patients with sporadic adrenocortical tumors. *Cancer Res* 2001; 61: 6762-7.

Gicquel C, Teinturier C, Gaston V, Brugiere L, Le Bouc Y. Adrenocortical tumors in childhood: incidence of tumor-predisposing syndrome and prognostic evaluation of molecular markers. *Horm Res* 2002; 58 (suppl 2): 145.

Godil MA, Atlas MP, Parker RI, Priebe CJ, Zerah MM, Kane P, et al. Metastatic congenital adrenal cortical carcinoma: a case report with tumor remission at 3 1/2 years. *J Clin Endocrinol Metab* 2000; 85: 3964-7.

Hawkins EP, Cagle PT. Adrenal cortical neoplasm in children. *Am J Clin Pathol* 1992; 98: 382-3.

Henry I, Grandjouan S, Couillin P, Barichard F, Huerre-Jeanpierre C, Glaser T, Philip T, Lenoir G, Chaussain JL, Junien C. Tumor-specific loss of 11p15.5 alleles in del11p13 Wilms tumor and in familial adrenocortical carcinoma. *Proc Natl Acad sci USA* 1989; 86: 3247-51.

Hoyme HE, Seaver LH, Jones KL, Procopio F, Crooks W, Feingold M. Isolated hemihyperplasia (hemihypertrophy): report of a prospective multicenter study of the incidence of neoplasia and review. *Am J Med Genet* 1998; 79: 274-8.

Kasat LS, Borwankar SS, Naregal A, Jain M. Complete spontaneous regression of a functioning adrenocortical carcinoma in an infant. *Pediatr Surg Int* 2001; 17: 230-1.

Keegan CE, Hammer GD. Recent insights into organogenesis of the adrenal cortex. *Trends Endocrinol Metab* 2002; 13: 200-8.

Kleihues P, Schauble B, Hausen A, Esteve J, Ohgaki H. Tumors associated with p53 germline mutations: A synopsis of 91 families. *Am J Pathol* 1997; 150: 1-13.

Latronico AC, Pinto EM, Domenice S, Fragoso MC, Martin RM, Zerbini MC, et al. An inherited mutation outside the highly conserved DNA-binding domain of the p53 tumor suppressor protein in children and adults with sporadic adrenocortical tumors. *J Clin Endocrinol Metab* 2001; 86: 4970-3.

Lefevre M, Gerard-Marchant R, Gubler JP, Chaussain JL, Lemerle J. Adrenal cortical carcinoma in children: 42 patients treated from 1958 to 1980 at Villejuif. In: Humphrey GB, Grindey GB, Dehner LP, Acton RT, Pysher TJ, eds. *Adrenal and endocrine tumors in children*, 1st ed. Boston: Martinus Nijhoff Publishers, 1983: 265-76.

Li FP, Fraumeni JF, Mulvihill JJ, Blattner WA, Dreyfus MG, Tucker MA, Miller RW. A cancer family syndrome in twenty-four kindreds. *Cancer Res* 1988; 48: 5358-62.

Liou LS, Kay R. Adrenocortical carcinoma in children: review and recent innovations. *Urol Clin North Am* 2000; 27: 403-21.

McFarlane DA. Cancer of the adrenal cortex: the natural history, prognosis and treatment in a study of fifty-five cases. *Ann R Coll Surg Engl* 1958; 23: 155-86.

McWhirter WR, Stiller CA, Lennox EL. Carcinomas in childhood. *Cancer* 1989; 63: 2242-6.

Malkin D, Li FP, Strong LC, Fraumeni JF, Nelson CE, Kim DH, *et al*. Germline p53 mutations in a familial syndrome of breast cancer, sarcomas, and other neoplasms. *Science* 1990; 250: 1233-8.

Mayer SK, Oligny LL, Deal C, Yazbeck S, Gagne N, Blanchard H. Childhood adrenocortical tumors: Case series and reevaluation of prognosis- A 24-year experience. *J Pediatr Surg* 1997; 32: 911-5.

Medeiros LJ, Weiss LM. New developments in the pathologic diagnosis of adrenal cortical neoplasms. *Am J Clin Pathol* 1992; 97: 73-83.

Michalkiewicz E, Sandrini R, Figueiredo B, Miranda ECM, Caran E, Oliveira-Filho AG, *et al*. Clinical and outcome characteristics of children with adrenal cortical tumors: A report from the International Pediatric Adrenal cortical Tumor Registry. *J Clin Oncol* 2004; 22: 838-45.

Pinto EM, Billerbeck AE, Villares-Fragoso MC, Mendonca BB, Latronico AC. Deletion mapping of chromosome 17 in benign and malignant adrenocortical tumors associated with the Arg337His mutation of the p53 tumor suppresor protein. *J Clin Endocrinol Metab* 2005; 90: 2976-81.

Ribeiro RC, Sandrini R, Schell M, Lacerda L, Sambiao GA, Cat I. Adrenal cortical carcinoma in children, a study of 40 cases. *J Clin Oncol* 1990; 8: 67-74.

Ribeiro RC, Sandrini F, Figueiredo B, Zambetti GP, Michalkiewicz E, Lafferty AR, *et al*. An inherited p53 mutation that contributes in a tissue-specific manner to pediatric adrenal cortical carcinoma. *Proc Natl Acad Sci USA* 2001; 98: 9330-5.

Ribeiro RC, Figueiredo B. Childhood adrenocortical tumors. *Eur J Cancer* 2004; 40: 1117-26.

Sabbaga CC, Avilla SG, Schulz C, Garbers JC, Blucher D. Adrenal cortical carcinoma in children: Clinical aspects and prognosis. *J Pediatr Surg* 1993; 28: 841-3.

Sandrini R, Ribeiro RC, DeLacerda L. Childhood adrenal cortical tumors. *J Clin Endocrinol Metab* 1997; 82: 2027-31.

Saracco S, Abramowsky C, Taylor S, Silverman RA, Berman BW. Spontaneously regressing adrenocortical carcinoma in a newborn: a case report with DNA ploidy analysis. *Cancer* 1988; 62: 507-11.

Stewart JN, Flageole H, Kavan P. A surgical approach to adrenocortical tumors in children: The mainstay of treatment. *J Pediatr Surg* 2004; 39: 759-63.

Stiller CA. International variations in the incidence of childhood carcinomas. *Cancer Epidemiol Biomarkers Prev* 1994; 3: 305-10.

Sullivan M, Boileau M, Hodges CV. Adrenal cortical carcinoma. *J Urol* 1978; 120: 660-5.

Teinturier C, Pauchard MS, Brugières L, Landais P, Chaussain JL, Bougnères PF. Clinical and prognostic aspects of adrenal cortical neoplasms in childhood. *Med Pediatr Oncol* 1999; 32: 106-11.

Varley JM, McGown G, Thorncroft M, James LA, Margison GP, Forster G, *et al*. Are there low-penetrance TP53 alleles? Evidence from chidhood adrenocortical tumors. *Am J Hum Genet* 1999; 65: 995-1006.

Weiss LM, Medeiros LJ, Vickery ALJ. Pathologic features of prognostic significance in adrenocortical carcinoma. *Am J Surg Pathol* 1989; 13: 202-6.

Wiedemann H. Complexe malformatif familial avec hernie ombilicale et macroglossie, un "syndrome nouveau". *J Genet Hum* 1964; 13: 223.

Wiedemann H. Tumors and hemihypertrophy associated with Wiedemann-Beckwith syndrome. *Eur J Pediatr* 1983; 141: 129.

Wieneke JA, Thompson LDR, Heffess CS. Adrenal cortical neoplasms in the pediatric population. A clinical and immunophenotypic analysis of 83 patients. *Am J Surg Pathol* 2003; 27: 867-81.

Wilkin F, Gagné N, Paquette J, Oligny L, Deal C. Pediatric adrenal cortical tumors: molecular events leading to insulin-like growth factor II gene overexpression. *J Clin Endocrinol Metab* 2000; 85: 2048-56.

Wolthers OD, Cameron FJ, Scheimberg I, Honour JW, Hindmarsh PC, Savage MO, *et al*. Androgen secreting adrenal cortical tumors. *Arch Dis Child* 1999; 80: 46-50.

Printed and bound by Corlet, Imprimeur, S.A.
14110 Condé-sur-Noireau
Printer's N°: 91788 - Copyright deposit: September 2006

Printed in France